The Hospital of Incurable Madness
L'hospedale de' pazzi incurabili (1586)

Medieval and Renaissance
Texts and Studies

Volume 352

Arizona Studies in the
Middle Ages and the Renaissance

Volume 26

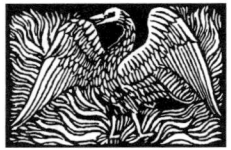

THE HOSPITAL OF INCURABLE MADNESS
L'HOSPEDALE DE' PAZZI INCURABILI (1586)

by
TOMASO GARZONI

Translation and Notes by
DANIELA PASTINA AND JOHN W. CRAYTON

Introduction by
MONICA CALABRITTO

ACMRS
(Arizona Center for Medieval and Renaissance Studies)
Tempe, Arizona
in collaboration with
BREPOLS
2009

HOSPITAL
OF INCURABLE
MADNESS

NEWLY CREATED
& brought to light by Thomaso Garzoni
of Bagnacavallo.

WITH THREE POEMS IN TERZA RIMA
on Madness
AT THE END.

TO THE EXCELLENT PHYSICIAN, AND
Illustrious Philosopher Signor Bernardino Paterno.

WITH PRIVILEGE

VENICE,
Giovanni Battista Somascho.
M.D.LXXXVI.

L'HOSPIDALE
DE' PAZZI
INCVRABILI

NVOVAMENTE FORMATO,
& posto in luce da THOMASO GARZONI
da Bagnacauallo.

CON TRE CAPITOLI IN FINE
sopra la Pazzia.

ALL'ECCELLENTISSIMO MEDICO, ET
Filosofo Chiarissimo Il Signor Bernardino Paterno.

CON PRIVILEGIO.

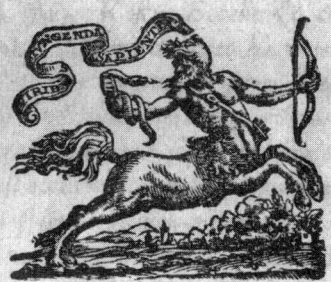
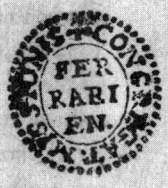

IN VENETIA,
Appresso Gio. Battista Somascho.
M. D. LXXXVI.

© Copyright 2009
Arizona Board of Regents for Arizona State University
and Brepols Publishers, n.v., Turnhout, Belgium

ASMAR Volume 26: ISBN 978-2-503-52895-3   D/2009/0095/78

Library of Congress Cataloging-in-Publication Data

Garzoni, Tomaso, 1549?-1589.
  [Ospidale de' pazzi incurabili. English]
  The hospital of incurable madness = L'hospedale de' pazzi incurabili (1586) / by Tomaso Garzoni ; translation and notes by Daniela Pastina and John W. Crayton ; introduction by Monica Calabritto.
       p. cm. -- (Medieval and Renaissance texts and studies ; v. 352) (Arizona studies in the Middle Ages and the Renaissance ; v. 26)
  Includes bibliographical references.
  ISBN 978-0-86698-400-3
  1. Psychiatry--Early works to 1900. I. Pastina, Daniela. II. Crayton, John W. III. Title. IV. Title: Hospedale de' pazzi incurabili.

RC340.G3213 2004
616.89--dc22
                                                                                    2009006748

∞
This book is made to last.
It is set in Adobe Caslon Pro,
smyth-sewn and printed on acid-free paper
to library specifications.
Printed in the United States of America

Table of Contents

Introduction	1
Dedication to Signor Bernardino Paterno	36
Dedicatory Poems by Policriti	38
Author's Prologue to the Spectators	41
Universal Madness	45
The Frenetic or Delirious — Minerva	55
The Melancholic and Savage — Jupiter	61
The Lazy and Good-for-Nothing — Apollo	67
The Drunkards — Abstemius	71
The Forgetful and Demented — Charon	77
The Dumb, Vacant, and Lifeless — Sentinius	81
The Round-Headed, Gross, and Simple-Minded — Ox of Egypt	85
The Idiots and Airheads — Samian Ewe	89
The Jerks and Giddies — Bubona	93
The Clumsy and Fatuous — Fatuellus	97
The Perverts — Themis	101
The Spiteful and Tarot Types — Nemesis	105
The Ridiculous — Risius	109

The Vainglorious —Juno	113
The Fakers and Jokers —Mercury	121
The Lunatics or Episodic Crazies—Hecate	125
The Love-Mad—Cupid	129
The Desperate—Venilia	137
The Heteroclites, the Odd, the Lame-Brained, and the Done-For—Vulcan	141
The Buffoons—Fabulanus	145
The Merry, Sweet, Facetious, and Loving—Bacchus	149
The Capricious and Frenzied —Tisifone	153
The Violent and Beastly: In Need of Ropes and Chains—Mars	157
The Over-the-Top and Triple-Refined —Volutina	161
The Obstinate, Like a Mule —Minos	165
The Hairless—Rhadamanthus	169
The Unbridled, Like a Horse—Hippona	173
The Extravagant, Extreme, and Witless—Hercules	177
The Diabolical: Those-Deserving-of-the-Gallows-a-Thousand-Times-Over—Pluto	183
On Madness in Women	189
Three Poems on Madness	
Poems by Theodoro Angelucci to Tomaso Garzoni: *On Madness*	201
In Praise of Madness by Signor Guido Casoni	211
To Angelucci: In Praise of Madness by the Author	217
Bibliography	225
Index	237

Introduction

Tomaso Garzoni's *L'hospedale* and Erasmus's *Praise of Folly*

L'hospedale de' pazzi incurabili, printed for the first time in Venice in 1586, is Tomaso Garzoni's "best-selling" compilation of a wide range of social deviance—from that caused by physiological illness, to anti-social behavior, to heresy. For Garzoni, madness must be considered the opposite of sanity, reason, and normality—a far cry from the all-inclusive vision of madness in Erasmus's *The Praise of Folly*. Following Paul's interpretation[1] of the figure of Christ as "fool," in the *Praise of Folly* (first printed in 1511) Erasmus had investigated the image of "wise" madness or "foolish" wisdom and praised Christ's followers as "fools."[2] In Italy, the *Praise of Folly* certainly influenced the author of *La pazzia*, a text commonly attributed to Vianesio Albergati, and Giuseppe Orologi, author of *L'inganno*.[3] Garzoni did not integrate Neo-Platonism and Christian religion as

---

[1] 1 Corinthians 1:25, 3:19, 4:10.

[2] For Erasmus's notion of madness, see M. A. Screech, "Good Madness in Christendom," in W. F. Bynum, Roy Porter, and M. Shepherd, eds., *The Anatomy of Madness. Essays in the History of Psychiatry, Vol. I: People and Ideas* (London and New York: Tavistock Publications, 1985), 25–39; Donald Gwynn Watson, "Erasmus' *Praise of Folly* and the Spirit of Carnival," *Renaissance Quarterly* 32 (1979): 333–53; Carlo Ossola, "Métaphore et inventaire de la folie dans la littérature italienne du XVIe siècle," in *Folie et déraison à la Renaissance: Colloque international tenu en novembre 1973 sous les auspices de la Fédération Internationale des Instituts et Sociétés pour l'étude de la Renaissance* (Brussels: Editions de l'Université de Bruxelles, 1976), 171–96.

[3] Erasmus's text, printed in Italy around 1515, was translated around the end of the 1530s. The book was included in the *Index librorum prohibitorum*, which was created in 1559. For an analysis of the influence of Erasmus's ideas in sixteenth-century Italy, see Silvana Seidel Menchi, *Erasmo in Italia: 1520–1580* (Turin: Bollati Boringhieri, 1987). In *La pazzia* (Venice: Valvassori, 1541), Albergati writes that the text belongs to the genre of the paradoxical praise, which was very common in the sixteenth century, and that madness "alone governs us, alone casts away from us the harsh anxieties and the heavy afflictions; she alone makes men and women satisfied and happy, who otherwise would be always miserable." For biographical information on Albergati, see *Dizionario biografico degli italiani* (Rome: Istituto della Enciclopedia Italiana, 1960), 1:621–24. In *L'inganno* (Venice: Giolito di Ferrara, 1562) Orologi considers the world "a mountain of

Erasmus did in his thought, since he belonged to a more orthodox religious current influenced by the decisions of the post-Tridentine Church and was willing to exalt wisdom, erudition, and common sense rather than the notion of *docta ignorantia* and "good" madness promoted by the more unorthodox elements of the Catholic world during the sixteenth century. However, Garzoni imitated the Erasmian tradition of madness when he wrote a poem praising folly in response to one composed by Teodoro Angelucci.[4] The two poems, along with another by Guido Casoni on the same subject, constituted the paratext of the first edition of *L'hospedale* printed in Venice, which Garzoni dedicated to a friend, the physician Bernardino Paterno.[5] Garzoni's poem has been considered an exercise

---

madness" (3) and assimilates wisdom to madness and vice versa (169–71). See also Paolo Cherchi, *Enciclopedismo e politica della riscrittura: Tomaso Garzoni* (Pisa: Pacini, 1980), 84. Shortly before 1523 Faustino Perisauli, known also by the name of Pier Saulo Faustino di Tredozio, wrote *De triumpho stultitiae*, a text influenced by Erasmus's *Praise of Folly*. See Angelo Scarpellini, "Erasmo e i letterati Romagnoli del Cinquecento," *Studi Romagnoli* 18 (1967): 369–90.

[4] Teodoro Angelucci, born in Belforte (Marche), was active as a physician and a man of letters in the second half of the sixteenth century, in Padua and Venice. He died around 1600. Angelucci composed medical treatises like *Ars medica* (Venice, 1588) and a series of polemical works against the Neo-Platonic philosopher Francesco Patrizi, of which *Quod metaphysica sint eadem quae physica* (1584) was the first to be printed. He translated Virgil's *Aeneid*. For further information about Angelucci, see *Dictionnaire des Sciences Médicales: Biographie Médicale* (Angelucci, Teodoro). For information about the polemic between Patrizi and Angelucci, see Martin Mulsow, "Ambiguities of the *Prisca Sapientia* in Late Renaissance Humanism," *Journal of the History of Ideas* 65 (2004): 1–13. For the possibility that Garzoni knew Erasmus's texts, or was at least acquainted with a *produzione filo-erasmiana*, see S. Barelli, ed., *Tomaso Garzoni: L'ospidale de' pazzi incurabili* (Rome: Antenore, 2004), "Introduzione," xxxvi–xxxvii.

[5] Guido Casoni was born in Serravalle (Treviso) in 1561 and died in 1625. A student of Girolamo Mercuriale in Padua, Casoni practiced medicine and cultivated his literary interests by founding four academies. He was strongly opposed to "Galileo's heresy." See *Dizionario biografico degli italiani* (*DBI*) for further biographical information. Both Casoni and Angelucci wrote dedicatory sonnets to Garzoni when *La piazza di tutte le professioni del mondo* was printed in 1585. The first edition of *L'hospedale* was printed in 1586 by Somasco in Venice (in 4°), by Cagnacini in Ferrara (in 12°), and by Bazachi in Piacenza (in 8°). Barelli (*L'ospidale*, lxxx) states that the Piacenza edition is clearly a reprint, presumably printed six months after those in Venice and Ferrara. In the Venice edition the three poems were placed at the end of the book. For the friendship between Garzoni and Paterno see Cherchi, *Enciclopedismo*, 10. Bernardino Paterno (15?-1592) taught medical theory in Pisa, Pavia, and Padua, where he lived from 1563 to 1592, the year he died. His works include *Explanationes in primam seu primi Canonis Avicennae* (Venice: De Franceschi, 1596) and *De humorum purgatione circa morborum initia tentanda* (Rome: Valerium Doricum, 1547). See *Dictionnaire des Sciences Médicales: Biographie Médicale* ("Paterno, Bernardino") and Nancy Siraisi, *Avicenna in Renaissance Italy: The Canon and Medical*

in the style which imitates the paradoxical praise of objects and activities, a very fashionable genre in sixteenth-century Italian literature.[6] While it is true that Garzoni's poem belongs to such a tradition, it is also valid to argue that such a composition creates a dialogue with Angelucci's poem and is an example of a different way of looking at madness from that shown in *L'hospedale*.[7]

In his poem Angelucci represents madness as inborn in human nature. In lines that remind the reader of the words pronounced by the chorus at the end of the first act of Tasso's *Aminta*, Angelucci writes that "to live loosely, and like a real madman, is more natural to man than to have his spirit convoluted by many rules," while honesty "is nothing but a fine illusion of vain and idle poets."[8] Furthermore, artists—poets, musicians, and painters—are inspired by madness, and Angelucci declares himself to be one of them. His allusions to Ariosto's *Orlando Furioso* and Petrarch's *Canzoniere* link his poem to the literary canon.[9] Angelucci's all-encompassing vision of madness is in stark contrast with Garzoni's notion of madness in *L'hospedale*, which separates the sane—the narrator, the reader—from the mad people. In his poem Garzoni adopts a vision of madness that reflects that expressed by Angelucci; however, he relies on himself to write about universal madness, and he uses popular literature and culture, rather than finding inspiration in the Muses and in literary canonical texts. Garzoni's role is not that of an inspired, frenzied author but that of a mountebank who entices his public. Among the names Garzoni mentions in his composition are those of the sixteenth-century empiric Leonardo Fioravanti, and of the writers Luigi Pulci and Teofilo Folengo, who elaborated popular language and tones into traditional poetic forms, content, and style through parody.[10] While Garzoni sings

---

Teaching in Italian Universities after 1500 (Princeton: Princeton University Press, 1987), 141 note 37 and *passim* for further biographical references and for an analysis of Paterno's position within the medical milieu of the period.

[6] Cherchi, *Enciclopedismo*, 122 and idem, "L'encomio paradossale nel manierismo," *Forum Italicum* 9 (1975): 368–84. Garzoni used the paradoxical praise again in a later work, *Il mirabile cornucopia consolatorio*, printed posthumously in 1601.

[7] For a reading of the three poems, see Valerio Marchetti, "La rappresentazione cinquecentesca della follia: un biblioteca senza archivio," in *La follia, la norma, l'archivio: Prospettive storiografiche e orientamenti archivistici*, ed. M. Galzigna (Venice: Marsilio, 1984), 161–69 and Barelli, "Introduzione," xli–xlvi.

[8] Angelucci's poem, 204 and 205.

[9] When he writes about love madness, Angelucci's words "Qual esser può più maledetta pania / di quella, ove se alcuno mette il piede / la dolce libertà per sempre impania," allude to lines 1–4 in canto 24.1 of the *Orlando Furioso*. One of the final lines of Angelucci's poem, which describes the lunatic's behavior ("di pensier in pensier sin quando ei dorme"), echoes the first line of Petrarch's sonnet 129 ("Di pensier in pensier, di monte in monte").

[10] For an analysis of Garzoni's use of Fioravanti's work in *La piazza universale di tutte le professioni del mondo* (1585), see Elvinia Vidali Giorio, "Una fonte del Garzoni: *Dello*

"in madness . . . / Of the humors and frenzies / That reside in all of our brains"[11] ("mattescamente humori, e frenesie, / ch'albergan nel cervel di tutti noi"), he does it by demoting madness from a form of divine inspiration linked to canonical literature to a phenomenon linked to popular tradition and parodic and comic literature. Garzoni's poem expresses an attitude towards madness that combines the topos of universal madness with popular literature and medicine within the theatrical frame of the mountebank's stage. These elements can be found in *L'hospedale*, with the exception of the notion of universal madness. In its place a strict distinction between sanity and madness tinges the entire text with strong moral overtones.

Tomaso Garzoni: biographical and historical context

From a short biography printed after Tomaso's death by his brother, Bartolomeo Garzoni, we learn that Tomaso was born as Ottaviano Garzoni to Pietro Garzoni and Altabella Lunardi in 1549 in Bagnacavallo, a small town in the province of Ravenna, then part of the Este dukedom.[12] Garzoni first studied letters; then, at fourteen, he studied law for three years in Ferrara and in Siena.[13] In 1566 Ottaviano entered, with the name of Tomaso, the order of the Regular Lateran Canons, which had one of their most important canonries in the church of Santa Maria in Porto in Ravenna. Since the beginning of the twelfth century the Church of Santa Maria in Porto followed the "regola portuense," an elaboration of the original rule of Saint Augustine, based on communal life and the rejection of property, which other canonries in and outside Italy adopted. In 1419, Obizzone da Polenta, lord of Ravenna, called the canonical community of S. Maria di Fregionaia near Lucca to restore new life to the languishing congregation of Santa Maria in Porto in order to check the decline that affected the congregation and the church in the thirteenth century. In 1421 Pope Martin V unified various

---

specchio di scientia universale di Leonardo Fioravanti," *Lingua nostra* 30 (1969): 39–43.

[11] "In Praise of Madness," 55–57, 212.

[12] Bartolomeo Garzoni, *Laconismo vitale circa l'autore*. The text is included as a preface to Tomaso Garzoni's *Serraglio de gli stupori del mondo* (Venice: Ambrogio Dei, 1613), his last work, published posthumously by his brother. The *Serraglio* has been reprinted in 2004 (Ravenna: Russi, 2004) with an introduction by Paolo Cherchi. See also *Dizionario biografico degli Italiani*, s.v. "Garzoni, Tomaso." In the documents "Atti dei notai del comune di Bagnacavallo" and "Governatori di Bagnacavallo" at the State Archive of Ravenna, Ada Sangiorgi was able to find some information about Garzoni's family going back three generations, which she submitted in a manuscript document to the organizers of the exhibit "Thomaso Garzoni e il suo tempo" which took place in Bagnacavallo in 1990. I was able to make reproductions of the document.

[13] Tomaso Garzoni, *Opere*, ed. Paolo Cherchi (Ravenna: Longo, 1993), 410–11 and *Dizionario biografico degli Italiani*, s.v. "Garzoni, Tomaso."

canonical Italian communities, including Santa Maria in Porto, under the congregation of Santa Maria in Fregionaia, which was later called "of the Salvatore Lateranense" by Pope Eugenius IV in a bull issued in 1445.[14] When Garzoni entered the order, the community of Santa Maria in Porto was one of the largest in northern Italy, with fifty individuals.[15] The members of the order followed the religious movement of the *devotio moderna* and, in accordance with the new decrees established by the Council of Trent, a renewed apostolic life, which also included pastoral activity.[16] Tomaso died at forty in 1589 in his native Bagnacavallo, where he had been called to preach on the Sacred Scriptures.[17]

From the dedicatory letters, the numerous sonnets dedicated to him, and the abundant citations in his texts, Garzoni seemed to have had direct contacts with or, at least, known very well the work of several Italian writers and intellectuals, such as the theologian Celso Mancini and Cipriano Giambelli, both belonging to the Lateran Canons, the humanist Fabio Paolini, the Jewish engineer and inventor Abramo Colorni, the musician Orazio Vecchi, the lawyer and writer Guido Casoni, the physician and man of letters Bartolomeo Burchelati, the poet Marco Stecchini, and the composer and writer Giuseppe Policreti.[18]

---

[14] For a detailed history of the Order of the Regular Lateran Canons, see *Dizionario degli Istituti di perfezione* (Rome: Edizioni Paoline, 1974–2003), s.v. "Canonici regolari," 46–154, and particularly 103–7 and 147–48. See also Tomaso Garzoni, *La Piazza universale di tutte le professioni del mondo*, ed. Paolo Cherchi and Beatrice Collina (Turin: Einaudi, 1996), 123–25; Ivan Simonini, "Tomaso Garzoni, uno zingaro in convento," in *Tomaso Garzoni: Uno zingaro in convento. Celebrazioni garzoniane, IV centenario (1589–1989), Ravenna-Bagnacavallo 1989–1990* (Ravenna: Longo, 1990), 9–25, here 10, and D. Luigi Lo Schiavo, "Tomaso Garzoni C.R.L. e la sua congregazione (1549–1589)," in *Tomaso Garzoni*, 27–34, here 29.

[15] Lo Schiavo, "Congregazione," 30.

[16] Lo Schiavo, "Congregazione," 32.

[17] On the reason why Garzoni was called to preach on the Sacred Scriptures in Bagnacavallo, see Giuseppe Ferretti, "L'umanista Tomaso Garzoni, religioso e scrittore Bagnacavallese nel quarto centenario della morte," *Torricelliana: Bollettino della società torricelliana di scienze e lettere* 41 (1990): 191–200. See also B. Collina, "Un 'cervello universale'," in *Tomaso Garzoni*, LXXII-CVII for Garzoni's activity as a preacher in northern Italy.

[18] For biographical information about Colorni, Burchiellati, Groto, and Guazzo see *Dizionario biografico degli Italiani*. Burchiellati, Colorni, and Groto wrote dedicatory sonnets for Garzoni's *La piazza*. For Celso Mancini, see Cherchi, "Introduzione," Garzoni, *Opere*, ed. idem (Ravenna: Longo, 1993), 8; Collina, "Un 'cervello universale'," Garzoni, *La Piazza* (Turin: Einaudi, 1996), LXXIV; for Fabio Paolini, see Gian Giuseppe Liruti, *Notizie delle vite ed opere scritte da letterati del Friuli* (Bologna: Forni, 1971), 3:352–72; Cherchi, Garzoni, *Opere*, 8; and Remo Avesani, "La professione dell' 'umanista' nel Cinquecento," *Italia medievale e umanistica* 13 (1970): 205–32; for Marco Stecchini, see Collina, "Un 'cervello'," XCI; for Policreti's musical activity, Giuseppe Gerbino, "The Madrigal and its Outcasts: Marenzio, Giovannelli, and the Revival of Sannazaro's *Arcadia*,"

He also seemed to have spent periods of time in Treviso, where he wrote part of *L'hospedale*, and in Ferrara, where he met Luigi Groto and Torquato Tasso, who both wrote sonnets dedicated to Garzoni for *La piazza di tutte le professioni del mondo* which was first printed in 1585.[19]

Between 1583 and 1589 he wrote a considerable number of texts, but he signed only those of explicit religious content, mostly written in Latin, as a member of the Regular Lateran Canons.[20] In the *Bibliotheca Selecta* the Jesuit Antonio Possevino saved only Garzoni's *Le vite delle donne illustri, e laide delle Sacre Scritture* (Venice, 1586) from censorship, while he harshly censored *La piazza di tutte le professioni del mondo* along with his other texts in the vernacular.[21] In his monumental work, written in Latin for the Catholic aristocracy, Possevino catalogued

---

Journal of Musicology 21 (2004): 3–41. For a short overview of the intellectual contacts Garzoni had in several Italian cities, see Collina, "Un 'cervello'," XCV-XCVII.

[19] Garzoni wrote from Treviso the dedicatory letter to Bernardino Paterno that appears in the Venice edition. See Adeline Charles Fiorato, "La folie universelle, spectacle burlesque et instrument idéologique dans *L'hospedale* de Tomaso Garzoni (1586)," in *Visages de la folie (1500–1600): Colloque tenu à la Sorbonne le 8 et le 9 mai*, ed. A. Redondo et A. Rochon (Paris: Publications de la Sorbonne, 1981), 31–45, here 31. For Angelo Groto, see *Dizionario biografico degli Italiani*. Garzoni dedicated *La piazza* to Alfonso II d'Este and *Le vite delle donne illustri della scrittura sacra* (Venice, Domenico Imberti, 1586) to Margherita d'Este Gonzaga, his wife. For an analysis of *Le vite*, see the introduction to the most recent edition of this work by Beatrice Collina: Garzoni, *Le vite* (Ravenna: Longo, 1994), 7–71.

[20] The texts which Garzoni signed as a member of the Regular Lateran Canons were his short treatise, *Le vite*; a translation of the Latin work of the mystical theologian Dionysius the Carthusian (1402/1403–1471), *Colloquio, overo dialogo del giudicio particolare dell'animo dopo la morte* (Venice, 1583); the edition of Hugh of Saint Victor's work in three volumes (*Hugonis de Sancto Victore, Canonici Regularis Lateranensis, tum pietate, tum doctrina insignis, Opera tribus tomis digesta* [Venice, 1588]); and *L'huomo astratto*, a discussion on the notion of natural ecstasy posthumously published in 1601. See also Bartolomeo Garzoni, *Laconismo*, b1. For an analysis of *L'huomo astratto* see Armando Maggi, "The Concept of 'natural ecstasy' in Tomaso Garzoni's *L'huomo astratto*," *Modern Philology* 101 (2003): 259–77.

[21] For Possevino's condemnation of *La piazza* see Antonio Possevino, *Bibliotheca Selecta* (Rome, 1593), 1:90–91, and Collina, "Un 'cervello universale'," XCI-XCII. For Possevino's negative judgment on the majority of Garzoni's texts in vernacular, see Antonio Possevino, *Apparatus sacer ad Scriptores Veteris et Novi Testamenti* (Venice, 1603) and Collina, "Un 'cervello universale'," XCI and n. 66. Possevino's *Bibliotheca* was considered the "more or less official model for the culture of the Counter Reformation": Gennaro Savarese and Andrea Gareffi, eds., *La letteratura delle immagini nel Cinquecento* (Rome: Bulzoni, 1980), 22–23. Antonio Possevino worked on the *Bibliotheca Selecta* for more than twenty years. See also Albano Biondi, "Aspetti della cultura cattolica post-tridentina: Religione e controllo sociale," in *Storia d'Italia, Annali 4: Intellettuali e potere*, ed. Corrado Vivanti (Turin: Einaudi, 1981), 296–99.

the culture of his period according to the ideological principles that the Catholic Church established after the Council of Trent. Garzoni's texts were not considered edifying for the reformed Catholic intelligentsia, but they were certainly acceptable for a larger, vernacular public. Garzoni's mixture of genres, styles, and languages expressed a tendency to popularize the official culture and its tenets, without denying the dictates of the reformed Catholic Church for which Garzoni worked.

Indeed, Garzoni popularized the cultural views of Tridentine Italy and made them available to a large public. In Garzoni's *L'hospedale,* for instance, madness is medicalized and catalogued but also mocked and thus made innocuous by the laughter of the sane individuals, thus creating a clear distinction between those who are normal and obey social and cultural norms and those who do not, who are then confined in 'L'hospedale'. Conforming to norms is characteristic of post-Tridentine culture, and Garzoni exemplifies such characteristics in his treatment of madness.

The main subject of several of Garzoni's texts was the representation of deviance from the canons of "normality" that characterized the Catholic Reformation discourse—including rules of conduct, censorship, and ideological surveillance in sixteenth-century Italy. *Il Theatro dei vari e diversi cervelli mondani* (1583), *L'hospedale,* and *La sinagoga degli ignoranti* (1589) dwell on the aberrant to define the normal. In *Il Theatro* brain—"cervello"—is equated both to temperament, "temperamento," and intelligence or "ingegno."[22] Garzoni creates several categories of *cervelli*, which he judges and subdivides according to moral standards.[23] Ignorance in *La Sinagoga* and madness in *L' hospedale* are two other categories that Garzoni uses to lambaste what is deemed deviance. In *La Sinagoga* Garzoni establishes a *congregazione* of "simpletons, fools and bird-brains," from which "wisdom is excluded, intelligence banished, truth is rejected, virtue is confined, and where vice, which should stay in the den, sits at the stern and reigns and orders with absolute authority over all the powers of the soul" (382).[24] For Garzoni, ignorance is not only an intellectual lack but also and especially a moral sin, a vice that needs to be extirpated through erudition and *scientia*.[25] As a representative of the Catholic Reformation, Garzoni condemned intellectual heresy

---

[22] In the "Author's Prologue to the Spectators" Garzoni defines the term *cervello* by excluding the definition that doctors and philosophers have given of it, that is, the "first and main organ of human life, house of the rational soul and instrument and principle of all the animal virtues," and he qualifies it "as a specific temperament, judgment, thought, or characteristic of the brain": Garzoni, *Opere*, 49.

[23] "Discorso proemiale," in Garzoni, *Opere*, ed. Cherchi, 47–51.

[24] Page numbers in the introduction refer to Garzoni, *Opere*, ed. Cherchi.

[25] Cherchi, *Enciclopedismo*, 108. The Catholic Church considered Jews, whose place of worship was the synagogue, ignorant for not recognizing Jesus as the Messiah, thus attributing a moral and ideological meaning to the term "ignoranza."

as well as religious unorthodoxy. In *L' hospedale*, for instance, Garzoni places in the category of the "madmen stubborn like a mule" individuals who have shown excessive obstinacy and gone against the precepts of their superiors. Among the examples taken from ancient history Garzoni includes Julian the Apostate, persecutor of the Christians, and some tyrants famous for their cruelty. In the discourse dedicated to the "hairless madmen," who betrayed their friends or superiors and were severely punished for their actions, Garzoni lists the Huguenots who were slaughtered during the night of St. Bartholomew in 1572. The version of the events occurred during the St. Bartholomew's massacre given in *L' hospedale* is clearly pro-Catholic, as it tries to represent the Huguenots as dangerous betrayers, since they are portrayed as wanting to exterminate the royal house, thus justifying the massacre.[26]

Several of Garzoni's texts possess a performative dimension evident in the titles — *teatro*, *sinagoga*. This dimension is further emphasized by the fact that in both *L'hospedale* and *La Sinagoga* the subject of the text is shown to a public who is the object of instruction and education. The space of *L' hospedale* is structured as a hospital and a theater at the same time, where the patients are shown to a titillated public, so that the latter will become "wiser" by observing in the former a complete lack of reason.[27] A hospital, it is divided into two sections according to gender, one for madmen and the other for madwomen. Masculine madness is subdivided into twenty-nine *discorsi*, each portraying a different type of mental alienation, to which corresponds a much shorter discussion on feminine madness, organized in twenty-nine descriptive vignettes. Many examples crowd each category of masculine madness, while women are secluded in the remotest part of the imaginary building, along an endless corridor that opens on twenty-nine cells. In each of them only one woman is confined. A prayer to a pagan divinity at the end of each discourse alludes to the possibility of a recovery for the madmen, while mad women are not offered such an option.[28]

---

[26] See Fiorato, "La folie universelle," 144 and eadem, "Présentation," in Garzoni, *L'hospedale de' pazzi incurabili/L'hospital des fols incurables* (Paris: Champion, 2001), 21–25.

[27] For the public display of mad patients in Italy, see Filippo Maria Ferro, "Il gran teatro della Romana pietà," in *L'ospedale dei pazzi di Roma dai papi al' 900: Lineamenti di assistenza e cura a poveri e dementi*, ed. Franca Fedeli Bernardini (Rome: Dedalo, 1994), 2:27–39, here 32, and Alessandra Bonfigli and Franca Fedeli Bernardini, " 'Quella carità che si sol fare alli pazzi acciò venghi a recuperare la sanità': Gli esordi dell' ospedale di S. Maria della Pietà e la cura dei dementi," in *L' ospedale dei pazzi di Roma dai papi al' 900*, 2:41–56, here 49.

[28] While Garzoni invented some of the divinities, like the god Sentino, he consulted Lilio Gregorio Giraldi's *De deis gentium* for most of the pagan gods and their attributes. Giraldi's text is divided into headings dedicated to one god or goddess or groups of lesser divinities. For Garzoni's use of Giraldi's work see Fiorato, "Présentation," and Cherchi, ed. Garzoni, *Opere*, 16.

L'hospedale

Garzoni provided the reader with a hybrid text, a collage of several genres—medical, encyclopedic, and novelistic—that need to be recognized and analyzed in order to understand the content of *L'hospedale*. He used several portions from other texts with, or more often without, acknowledging the source. Far from being an isolated example, Garzoni illustrates the relationship writers had with the tradition in the second half of the sixteenth century.[29] In *L'hospedale* Garzoni juxtaposed the orthodox medical explanation of several kinds of madness with the popularized account of their causes. He exemplified the traditional categories of madness through quotations from medical texts but also with a long list of short stories or anecdotes that belong both to the "high" genre of the commonplace and to the "low" genre of popular witty stories or *facezie*. The anecdote narrates events with famous historical characters as protagonists, emphasizes the protagonists' moral qualities, such as virtues and vices, and helps the narrator strengthen his narration by referring to the tradition. Unlike the short narrative section in the medical treatise, which has a somewhat temporal dimension, the anecdote is taken out of its historical context and becomes one of the forms in which the *auctoritas* of the classics is expressed in later texts.[30] The *facezie* of the Tuscan country priest Arlotto Mainardi (1396–1484) were first transmitted orally, then collected by an anonymous compiler and printed for the first time in the first quarter of the sixteenth century. They are short stories which all have as their protagonist the *piovano* or parish priest Arlotto with his earthy witticisms. Garzoni quoted Arlotto several times in *L'hospedale* and puts him among the "pazzi allegri, sollazzevoli, faceti ed amorevoli" (Discourse XXII, p. 149) ("joyful, entertaining jesting and loving madmen"); he also quoted the buffoon Gonella, who lived in the fourteenth century and whose stories were narrated by Sacchetti

---

[29] See Cherchi, *Enciclopedismo*, esp. 1 and 139–40, and "Introduzione," Garzoni, *Opere* 18 on the notion of *riscrittura*. More recently, Cherchi has edited a collection of essays on this subject entitled *Sondaggi sulla riscrittura del Cinquecento* (Ravenna: Longo, 1998). For an analysis of the association among *riscrittura*, imitation, and memory, see L. Bolzoni, *La stanza della memoria* (Turin: Einaudi, 1995) esp. 65, 120, 195. See also Giancarlo Mazzacurati and Michel Plaisance, eds., *Scritture di riscritture: Testi, generi, modelli nel Rinascimento* (Rome: Bulzoni, 1987) and Luciana Borsetto, *Il furto di Prometeo: Imitazione, scrittura, riscrittura nel Rinascimento* (Alessandria: Edizioni dell' Orso, 1990), esp. 10–13. See also Garzoni, "Nuovo Prologo," in *La Piazza*, 32–40.

[30] P. Cherchi, "Invito alla lettura della *Piazza*," in Garzoni, *La Piazza*, ed. idem and B. Collina (Turin: Einandi, 1996), XLII. In *I marmi* (1552) Doni created a "concordance of historical facts" according to which the events are gathered together on the basis of their moral qualities, and not of their historical context. See Cherchi, *Enciclopedismo*, 23.

and Bandello and gathered in the collection *Facezie, motti, buffonerie et burle del Piovano Arlotto, del Gonella e del Barlachia* printed in Florence in 1568.[31]

To contain madness, Garzoni uses the hospital as a rhetorical device analogous to the encyclopedic notion of the *theatrum*, which stood for a vast work of encyclopedic nature and was linked to the *silva*, a very successful genre in the second part of the sixteenth century.[32] The *theatrum* is the opposite of the *silva*: while the latter shows the reader a disorderly subject matter, the *theatrum* organizes the *materia* into a harmonious universe.[33] The metaphor of the theater was also used to define "memory theaters," memory treatises that relied on ancient rhetoric and Neo-Platonic and Hermetic doctrines and organized knowledge and memory in spatial terms and imagery.[34] From the inner theater of memory, created with the help of mnemonic and rhetorical devices, to the bookish theater of the encyclopedic knowledge and rhetoric, the metaphor of the theater implies a public that is able to transform words into images and to visualize and consequently see the concept as performed before its eyes.[35]

Garzoni was aware of the rhetorical tradition of the theaters, since he dedicated a chapter to Raymon Lull and another to the "professori di memoria" in *La piazza*.[36] He also knew the various groups making up the medical hierarchy, but

---

[31] For Piovano Arlotto, see *Motti e facezie del Piovano Arlotto*, ed. Gianfranco Folena (Milan: Ricciardi, 1995 [1st ed. 1953]). Letterio di Francia writes that the *Facezie* attributed to Arlotto Mainardi were printed thirty-five times during the sixteenth century: Letterio di Francia, *Novellistica* (Milan: Vallardi,1925), 190–91. See Fiorato, ed., 314 n.509 for the figures of Gonella and Burlacchia.

[32] For an analysis of theatrical metaphors in the encyclopedic tradition see Ann Blair, *The Theater of Nature: Jean Bodin and Renaissance Science* (Princeton: Princeton University Press, 1997), 153–79. In *Enciclopedismo* Cherchi analyzes Garzoni's works in the context of the genre of the *theatrum*, which was very popular in sixteenth-century Europe. Relying on Bodin's definition of the term, Cherchi characterizes this genre as "mirror of nature and an encyclopedia that seeks to represent by reflection the divine majesty." See also Paolo Cherchi, "La selva rinascimentale: profilo di un genere," in *Ricerche sulle selve rinascimentali*, ed. idem (Ravenna: Longo Editore, 1999), 9–41. Relying on the definition of Pedro Mexía, the author of the first *silva* in vernacular (*Silva de varia lección* [1540]), Cherchi defines the term as "the disorderly disposition of the subject matter" (13).

[33] For an explanation of the relationship among *theatrum, silva,* and encyclopedia see Cherchi, *Enciclopedismo*, 31–35.

[34] Giulio Camillo's "theatre" is the most famous example of this genre. See Frances Yates, *The Art of Memory* (Chicago: University of Chicago Press, 1984 [1st ed. 1966]), 129–72. See also Lina Bolzoni, *Il teatro della memoria: Studi su G. Camillo* (Padua: Liviana, 1984) and idem, "Come costruire il tesoro della memoria: La tradizione mnemotecnica," in Cherchi, ed., *Ricerche sulle selve rinascimentali,* 166–69.

[35] Valerio Marchetti, "Tassonomie, citazioni, esempi e luoghi comuni," in *Tomaso Garzoni: Polyhistorismus und Interkulturalität in der frühen Neuzeit*, ed. Italo Michele Battafarano (Bern: Peter Lang, 1991), 9–25, here 22–23.

[36] *La piazza, discorsi* XXI and LX. See also Yates, *The Art of Memory*, 208–9.

one can only speculate that he knew the organization of the hospitals in Italy.[37] Within this context, the structure of *L'hospedale* is a space, alternative to that of the theater, that organizes knowledge and memory.[38] In this rhetorical space the narrator catalogues and selects his material. Garzoni's perception of the hospital and madness through his fictional construction affected his response to disease and, in general, to aberration. Garzoni seemed interested in exploring the medical and naturalistic dimension of madness, while still perceiving it from a moralistic point of view.[39]

From the first pages of the text the narrator presents the reader with an interesting mixture of languages, genres, and traditions. Medical terms and medical quotations are juxtaposed with mythological definitions, biblical allusions, and popular definitions of madness and mad individuals. The reader is also made immediately aware of a strong didactic component, exemplified in the narrator's moralistic notion of madness as an aberration to be punished, and a medical dimension underlined by the narrator's definition of madness. Garzoni used the medical tradition as one of the primary ways to legitimize his definition but also as a foil for the more vulgarized language about it. In the introductory discourse "on universal madness," madness is represented as a monstrous entity worse than the three-headed Geryon, which does not affect the narrator but transforms the subject deemed insane into an animal. While in Ariosto's *Orlando Furioso,* which Garzoni quotes several times in his text, madness and folly are usually comic and include the narrator, in Garzoni madness often produces a satirical and moralistic laughter that distances the narrator and the public even further from the mad person.[40] The narrator tries to domesticate and dissect madness in order to

---

[37] *La piazza*, discorsi VII, XVII, XXIII.

[38] Valerio Marchetti, "La rappresentazione della follia: una biblioteca senza archivio," in *La follia, la norma, l'archivio: Prospettive storiografiche e orientamenti archivistici*, ed. M. Galzigna (Venice: Marsilio, 1984), 136–49.

[39] Even if in *L'hospedale* there are no cases of madness caused by demonic possession, Garzoni classifies the last category of madness "of madmen deserving-of-the-gallows-a-thousand-times-over or diabolical madmen" and writes: "Nor is there a paucity of examples of this type, for the Devil goes everywhere, sowing his seeds, like weeds, and they spring forth, teeming, from themselves, like the Hydra; and with the flames of their iniquity, they set fire to heaven and earth" (p. 183). In *L'hospedale* Garzoni's description of madness is only generically connected to the existence of demonic powers, since it does not specify the extent to which demons are believed to possess human beings and make them act according to their will. Garzoni broaches the subject of the devil and witchcraft several times in *Il Serraglio de gli stupori del mondo* (Venice, 1613). I make no attempt to list a growing bibliography on early modern witchcraft and demonic possession, but see at least Stuart Clark, *Thinking with Demons: The Idea of Witchcraft in Early Modern Europe* (New York: Oxford University Press, 1997) and Matteo Duni, *Under the Devil's Spell. Witches, Sorcerers, and the Inquisition in Renaissance Italy* (Florence: SUF, 2007).

[40] See Ariosto, *Orlando Furioso*, 24.3.1–8.

distance himself and his audience from the perversion of reason exemplified by the patients in the hospital. However, the quasi-medical definition of madness turns into a colorful list of similes in which the behavior of a mad person is compared to that of a "mill hack" and his head to a "watermelon."[41]

The monsters to which the narrator compares madness—Cadmus' serpent, the Chimera, the dragon of the Hesperides, Corebus' monster, Geryon—make up a conflation of mythological images and produce a hellish vision. Some of these monstrous figures populate Dante's *Inferno*—Cadmus transformed into a serpent, the Minotaur, Geryon—expressing sins that are punished for eternity. The narrator follows the implication that madness is associated with moral sin by stating that it is a monstrous external force that ravishes people's minds and makes them believe they are wise when they are out of their minds. A few lines later, Garzoni conforms to the medical tradition of Galen and his followers by quoting (in a significantly modified way) an aphorism by Hippocrates and by having madness located in the brain and affecting the "imaginative" and "cogitative" faculties, traditionally considered the functions of the animal or rational soul.[42] Garzoni then imperceptibly slides into a list of risible images in which the mad individual is assimilated to a fruit and an animal, makes a biblical allusion, and concludes his presentation of universal madness by defining it as a phenomenon that puts everybody on the same level, regardless of social distinctions.[43]

The medical and the encyclopedic traditions: Altomare, Fernel, Tixier

Garzoni's *L'hospedale* is the product of the consultation of a few works, among which are the medical treatises by Donato Antonio Altomare and Jean Fernel, Jean Tixier de Ravisy's *Officina*, and Lilio Gregorio Giraldi's *De deis gentium* and

---

[41] "Once she enters the domain of the brain, she obfuscates the imagination, perverts thought, alienates the mind, corrupts reason, and so impedes a man that he cannot understand, choose, speak, nor do anything right, but instead, with troubled fantasies, a vacillating spirit, sick reasoning, a brain in agony, a head as vacuous as a dried-up watermelon, he wanders aimlessly, like a mill-horse, around a thousand sillinesses, as pitiable as he is ridiculous" (p. 46).

[42] According to Galen, the five functions of the rational or animal soul were imagination, judgment, memory, apperception, and movement, p. 47.

[43] "She does not spare kings, has no respect for emperors, holds no captain in esteem, does not consider the learned, pays no attention to the rich, has no fear of nobles, and has no regard that may stop her, striking a hailstorm of blows this way and that at all mortal offspring."

Vita Herculis.⁴⁴ Garzoni uses texts that were already collections of commonplaces and quotations in the medical and encyclopedic traditions as is the case with Tixier's *Officina* and Altomare's *De medendis*.⁴⁵

---

⁴⁴ Jean Fernel (1497–1558) was a renowned French physician. Vesalius was one of his pupils, Catherine de' Medici one of his patients. His *Medicina* (Paris: Wechel, 1554) included several of his earlier works—*De naturali parte medicinae* (1542), re-titled *Physiologia*, and *Therapeutica*—and a new text, *Pathologia*. After Fernel's death, Guillaume Plancy, his associate for ten years, edited Fernel's work, which was printed under the title of *Universa Medicina* (Paris, 1567). In the present study I refer to the 1554 edition of Fernel's *Medicina*. For further biographical information on Fernel see Jacques Roger, *Jean Fernel et les problèmes de la médicine de la Renaissance* (Paris: Palais de la découverte, 1960). The Neapolitan Donato Antonio Altomare (beginning of the sixteenth century-ca. 1562) taught at Naples and followed the school of Hippocrates and Galen, whom he constantly commented upon in his work *De medendis humani corporis malis. Ars medica* was printed for the first time in 1553 in Naples. For further biographical information see *Dizionario biografico degli Italiani*. In the present study I refer to the 1560 edition of *De medendis humani corporis malis* printed in Venice. Jean Tixier de Ravisy, known also under the Latin name of Ravisius Textor, was born around 1470. He studied at the Collège de Navarre in Paris and became a professor of rhetoric. The *Officina* was printed for the first time in 1520. The edition that I consulted for the present study was printed in Basel in 1552. For further biographical information on Tixier de Ravisy, see M. Mignon, *Études sur le théatre français et italien de la Renaissance* (Paris: Champion, 1923), 32–61; J. Vodoz, *Le théatre latin de Ravisius Tixier (1470–1524)* (Wintherthur: Imprimerie G. Ziegler, 1898); and Walter Ong, "Commonplace Rhapsody: Ravisius Textor, Zwinger and Shakespeare," in *Classical Influences on European Culture 1500–1700* (Cambridge: Cambridge University Press, 1976), 91–126. Lilio Gregorio Giraldi (1479–1552) followed the cardinal Rangone, bishop of Modena, to Rome in 1514 where he stayed until the sack of Rome in 1527, the year in which he lost his library and all his property. He found refuge in Modena in the service of Giovanni Francesco Pico della Mirandola, who was assassinated in 1533. After his death, Giraldi returned to his native city of Ferrara, where he died in 1548. For further biographical information see *Dizionario biografico degli Italiani*. The *De deis gentium* was first printed in Basel in 1548. The edition that I used in the present study was printed in Ferrara in 1563. Giraldi's *Life of Hercules* (*Vita Herculis*) was first published in 1539 (Basle: Michael Isingen). The copy of the *Vita Herculis* that I consulted is included in Giraldi's *Opera omnia* printed in Leiden in 1696. In his edition of Garzoni's *Opere* (1993) Cherchi identified the texts by Altomare, Fernel, Tixier, and Giraldi as sources that Garzoni used for the composition of *L' hospedale*. Garzoni also used many *Adagia* of Erasmus and substantial borrowings from Aulus Gellius's *Noctes Atticae* and Athenaeus's *Deipnosophistae*.

⁴⁵ Brasavola's *Aphorismorum Hippocratis et Galeni commentaria et annotationes* is another medical text Garzoni used in *L'hospedale*. For a list of sources that Garzoni used in his works see also Garzoni, *La piazza*, 16.

Altomare and Fernel

At the beginning of *L'hospedale* (discourses I-VI) Garzoni uses the medical authority of Donato Antonio Altomare and Jean Fernel. Altomare was a follower of Hippocrates and Galen, and, like many other representatives of Renaissance medical tradition, he conceived of his texts as a way to justify his positions and to discuss his take on the subject from a textual point of view.[46] While Altomare transforms Galen's case of a man who "is afraid that Atlas who supports the world will become tired and throw it away and he and all of us will be crushed and pushed together" (Discourse 3, p. 62) into a *sententia* to be cited as part of the textual tradition and no longer as a sample of direct observation,[47] Garzoni transforms Altomare's section into a short narrative that sounds more like a popular story than the example of ancient medical *experientia*.[48] Garzoni adds a few colorful particulars to the original story of Galen, like the fact that the patient, out of the fear caused by melancholy, could not stand up and would always walk backward, as if under the effect of the enormous weight of Mount Olympus. These additions can be considered an intrusion of popular elements, probably morsels of oral tradition, into the "high," official language of medical tradition.

---

[46] Humanist discoveries of ancient medical texts and the possibility of reading some of them in the original Greek allowed the medical community to 'rediscover' Hippocrates and Galen and to put their system in dialogue with the modern doctrine, which claimed to be based on observation and *experientia*. The Renaissance notion of *experientia* did not completely exclude the idea of experience, but was still based on bookish information or just simple hearsay.

[47] "Another man feared that Atlas, who is said to sustain the universe, oppressed by such a burden, would shake off the universe from him, that the universe would be dashed into pieces with him and that we too would perish with it" (Altomare, *Ars medica*, Caput VII). Renaissance physicians adopted Galen as their model. This process was facilitated by Galen himself, who would disseminate his writings with autobiographical anecdotes, with the intent of "exemplify[ing] the qualities that physicians ought to emulate." See Jerome Bylebyl, "Medicine, Philosophy, Humanism in Renaissance Italy," in John W. Shirley and David Hoeniger, eds., *Science and the Arts in the Renaissance* (London and Toronto: Associated University Presses, 1985), 27–49, here 39. See also Nancy Siraisi, *The Clock and the Mirror: Girolamo Cardano and Renaissance Medicine* (Princeton: Princeton University Press, 1997), 207.

[48] "Galen, among others, in the third book of his *On the Affected Parts*, describes a man who, imagining that he had become a total crock-pot, gave way to everyone he met, in order not to smash into them and hurt himself. And Altomare, in his treatise *Treatment of Diseases of the Human Body*, mentions two others: one, hearing a rooster crowing and beating its wings, he also flapped his arms and imitated the bird's crowing and flapping. The other one feared that Atlas —whom the poets say holds up Mount Olympus—might become tired of holding this huge weight and might throw it down and he would be crushed under the mountain" (Discourse III, "The Melancholic and Savage").

Garzoni follows Altomare's text rather faithfully when he defines lycanthropy and describes the effects of this illness on the physical appearance and on the mental faculties of the sick subject, but thoroughly elaborates a story of *insania lupina* or "wolf-madness" that Altomare has narrated in his treatise.[49] For Altomare, this story is meant to explain and exemplify to the reader how this type of madness modified the functioning of certain mental faculties:

> [...] Indeed, one day when this man, possessed by such affliction and before having met me, had come towards me, I moved away in fear, while he, looking at me a little, went away. With him there was a crowd of people and he was carrying on his shoulders a whole leg and the shin of a dead man. This man, cured at last, became free [of the illness]. When he ran into me again, he asked me why I was afraid, since I had come upon him in that place, while he was mad: from these [signs] it is clear that his memory had not been damaged.

Garzoni transforms Altomare's "clinical" story into a macabre vignette:

> ... and the rumor spread from person to person through all of the Jewish households, that this man had disinterred Master Simone (for this was the dead Jew's name) and he had created a wonderful Synagogue of Mirth in their presence, seeing that the madman had taken an arm-bone to use as a bat in his ball games and the body, full of disgusting liquid, for a ball. And with every blow, the soupy mixture spewed out. It took two weeks for the community just to quell the stench. Even the stingier types preferred to pay one *carlino*—it would have been too painful not to have the piazza cleaned up—rather than to breathe in Master Simone's perfume, which was no joking matter. (p. 63-4)

The stench of the liquid pouring from the corpse and the eccentric game that the madman plays with parts of the mutilated body in the square of a small town are the most peculiar and original elements of Garzoni's narration. Garzoni gives the

---

[49] Altomare describes with the following words the *signa* that mark an individual affected by the "wolf's madness": "[...] facies eorum pallida est: oculi sicci ad videndum imbecilli, et non lachrymantur, ipsorumque oculos cavos videbis: linguam siccam, et salivam omnino non profundunt. Sitis ipsis adest immodica [...]" (97) ("[...] their face is pale: they have dry, weak-sighted eyes which do not shed a tear. You will observe that their eyes are hollow, that their tongue is dry, since they do not produce saliva at all"). Altomare's account reminds the reader of the description of Orlando in canto 24 of the *Orlando Furioso*, at the moment of his fortuitous meeting with Angelica: "Quasi ascosi avea gli occhi ne la testa, / la faccia macra, e come un osso asciutta, / la chioma rabuffata, orrida e mesta, / la barba folta, spaventosa e brutta" (60. 1–4) ("[Orlando's] eyes were almost hidden in his head, his face was emaciated and dry as a bone, his hair was ruffled, bristly and melancholy; his beard was bushy, hideous and ugly").

protagonist of the story a name, Fornaretto, and a place of provenance—Lugo, in Emilia Romagna. Fornaretto unearths the body of an octogenarian Jewish man affected by dropsy, and begins playing ball with it, spreading the stench of the liquid that was within the corpse all around the Jewish community. By the time the reader has paused for a second to free himself from the repulsion that he may feel from reading this macabre scene, he almost forgets that the story reported is supposed to be an exemplum of *insania lupina*. The reader's attention is seized by the image of a mangled, smelly corpse and by the emphasis given to the identity of the dead man and of the people who were present at the odd scene. At the end of the story, Garzoni alludes to the infamous stereotype of Jewish greed. He also lets the reader infer the uncleanness of the Jews by pointing to the fact that it was only because the stench has been so unbearable that every Jew in the community decided to pay the penalty for cleaning the area from such a revolting smell. What started as an orthodox explanation of *lupinositas* progressed into an implicit attack on the Jewish community, made to look as odd as the madman.[50]

In the second discourse dedicated to the "frenzied and delirious madmen" Garzoni translates almost literally Jean Fernel's treatment of melancholy, frenzy, and delirium, but at the end he substitutes the popularized version of frenzy for the orthodox medical explanation that Fernel provides in his treatise:[51]

---

[50] I make no attempt to provide a full bibliography on the Jewish community in the early modern period, but see at least John G. Gager, *The Origins of Anti-Semitism: Attitudes toward Judaism in Pagan and Christian Antiquity* (New York: Oxford University Press, 1983); Anna Foa, *Ebrei in Europa: Dalla peste all'emancipazione* (Bari: Laterza, 1997); Robert Bonfil, *English Jewish Life in Renaissance Italy*, trans. Anthony Oldcorn (Berkeley: University of California Press, 1994); Michele Luzzati, Michele Olivari, and Alessandra Veronese, eds., *Ebrei e cristiani nell'Italia medievale e moderna: conversioni, scambi, contrasti: atti del VI congresso internazionale dell'AISG, S. Miniato, 4–6 novembre 1986* (Rome: Carucci, 1988); Adriano Prosperi, "La Chiesa e gli ebrei nell'Italia del' 500," in *Ebraismo e antiebraismo: immagine e pregiudizio* (Florence: Giuntina, 1989), 171–83.

[51] "[Madness] with fever is either frenzy or delirium. However, they are different since delirium alone is produced by the bile or by thin blood spreading through the brain, or by the warm exhalation of the stomach, the diaphragm, or the entire body, such as is aroused in the vigor of very strong fevers. Frenzy is always produced primarily by an affection of the brain, either inflammation or erysipelas. They also differ in that delirium is most of the time the symptom of fever or a more serious illness, while frenzy is not the symptom, but the cause of the fever. Furthermore, delirium is extremely frequent, while frenzy is very rare": Fernel, "Principis facultatis symptomata. Caput II" (127). "But physicians distinguish between frenzy and delirium, although both of them are associated with a fever, because delirium—as John Fernelius Ambianus in the fifth book of his medical works has written—is sometimes caused by bile and sometimes by an effusion of thin blood into the brain, and sometimes by other causes. But frenzy is always caused by that inflammation of the brain mentioned above. In addition, most of the time

Because I don't wish to speak about madness the way physicians do, but rather according to the plain talk of the people, I have subsumed both frenetic and delirious madness under one heading, because when one speaks *bus* and *bas* about something, we ordinarily say that he is speaking like a frenetic or delirious madman, since that person is undergoing the same experience as those who are properly afflicted by delirium or frenzy. (p. 66)

A few pages later (p. 61), in the third discourse dedicated to the "melancholic and savage madmen," Garzoni attributes to Fernel the definition of melancholy he uses in the text, while the sections that precede and follow the citation from Fernel's treatise derive from Altomare.[52] Garzoni starts the discourse in what might seem a very scientific tone, by claiming that many doctors, both ancient and modern, agree on the definition of melancholy and its symptoms.[53] The list of experts that Garzoni produces in support of his definition of melancholy, and which he attributes to Altomare, is a slightly elaborated translation of Altomare's text.[54]

---

delirium is a symptom of fever or some other more serious malady. However fever is not a symptom, but is the cause of frenzy. Delirium occurs fairly often, but frenzy is very rare. Frenzy is a far more violent illness than delirium": Garzoni, Discourse II, "The Frenetic or Delirious."

[52] "Melancholy is a certain type of delirium without fever, deriving prevalently from the melancholic humor, which has occupied the site of the mind [...] however, it is common to all melancholic individuals that their brain is affected either in substance or by agreement. In his investigation [of melancholy] Paulus [Aegineta] observed that the brain is affected in a state of melancholy. Galen has bequeathed this same doctrine before him in book three of *De locis affectis*": Altomare, *De medendis*, chapter VII (74). For Fernel's text, see Garzoni, *Opere*, 266, n. 1 and 2.

[53] "The general opinion of all learned physicians about that condition which we call Frenzy—and especially of Galen in the first of his *Prorrhetics*—is this [...]."

[54] "[...] melancholy should be considered a sort of delirium not associated with fever, which is caused by nothing else but an excess of melancholic humors which have occupied the seat of the mind. In fact, it is common to all melancholics that their brains are diseased, either essentially or by consensus, as Altomare states in the seventh chapter of his *Medicinal Art*. This is also Galen's opinion in the third book of his *On the Diseases and Symptoms of the Parts of the Body* and of Hippocrates in the sixth book of his *On Common Disorders*, and of Paulus Medicus in the fortieth chapter of his third book."

Tixier de Ravisy and Giraldi

Tixier's *Officina* was a repository of commonplace and encyclopedic knowledge published for the first time around 1520 and frequently reprinted until the end of the seventeenth century.[55] In a dedicatory letter to his former teacher Jean de Bulvac, Tixier claimed that the disposition and organization of the material was his, while the content of the *Officina* derived totally from other sources, so much that it resembled the "corneille d'Horace, toute revetue des plumes d'autrui" ("Horace's crow, all dressed up in the feathers of others").[56] By choosing the title *Officina* Tixier underlined the dimension of "laboratory" that the text was meant to have for his readers, young students of grammar and rhetoric. All the short anecdotes of the *Officina* are structured more or less in the same way. The name of a historical figure is associated with a quality—a virtue or a flaw, a vice—and it is followed by the name of the author from whom the information has been taken. The style is dry, and the narration is a gigantic sum of quotations the authority of which is attributed not to the text from which they are taken but to their author. The constant succession of quotations has the effect of engendering other quotations through aggregation. The brevity of the anecdotes allows also for the possibility of memorization.

After having used Altomare's and Fernel's definitions of melancholia in the third discourse, Garzoni narrates the story of Pisander that he has collected from Tixier's *Officina*.[57] Tixier's passage, which belongs to the section in the *Officina* dedicated to the "furious and insane people" and is itself a quotation, provides the rough material for Garzoni's longer elaboration.[58] Next to the citation from

---

[55] The titles of the seven chapters into which Tixier's *Officina* is divided are: "De deis eorumque cultu"; "De mundo"; "De tempore et eius partibus"; "De homine"; "De magistratu"; "De artibus liberalibus ac manuariis, item de variis etiam artificibus"; and "De variis virtutibus ac viciis."

[56] The crow image comes from Horace, *Epistles*, 3. Garzoni uses the same image to define borrowing in the prologue to *La piazza*. Cherchi uses the term "translation" to define the way Garzoni took material from the "officine umanistiche," like Tixier's work (*L' enciclopedismo*, 26–27). In *L' hospedale* Garzoni mentioned Tixier de Ravisy only once: "Johann Ravisio Textor puts among the ridiculous madmen also a certain Xenophantus [...]". For an analysis of Tixier's work, and particularly of the *Officina*, see Paolo Cherchi, "L'*Officina* del Testore e alcune opere di Ortensio Lando," *Modern Language Notes* 95 (1980): 210–19.

[57] "Pisander fell into such a state of madness that he feared running into his soul everywhere, because he thought that it had abandoned him (Celio, book 9, chapter 26)."

[58] "Celio, in the twenty-sixth chapter of his ninth book, lists a man named Pisander among this sort of madmen. Thinking that he had died, he became wondrously afraid of running into his own soul which he considered to be a mortal enemy of his body, and he was determined not to have anything to do with it, since it had treated him so badly and was so unfaithful in leaving him." See this edition, p. 62. Almost every discourse in

Tixier's text, Garzoni assembles a story that belongs to the popular tradition: "But what shall we say of Nicoletto da Gattia who, suffering this disposition of the brain, imagined that he had become a wick in an oil lamp and, for this reason, wanted everybody to blow on him before, behind and on the sides, fearing that if he burned too much he would vanish completely?" (62). In the space of a few lines three borrowings—Altomare, Fernel, and Tixier de Ravisy—succeed one after the other, showing no substantial difference among them. Garzoni equates the medical and the commonplace tradition by emphasizing their citational and anecdotic dimension.

Garzoni uses the index of Tixier's work to consult the headings or "places" that he thought were connected to a specific category of madness. For instance, when he creates a long list of vignettes from two sections of Tixier's *Officina*, which belong to two separate chapters, probably he has consulted the index first and then decided that elements from both entries could fit the discourse on *dementia*.[59] In general, Garzoni faithfully translates the entire passage from the *Officina*, but sometimes he enriches the story with particulars that are absent from the original.[60] Sometimes Garzoni employs the same headings for more than one discourse.[61]

Garzoni's method of consulting and elaborating Tixier's work emphasizes the encyclopedic nature of the *Officina* and the endless possibilities for elaborating its *materia*.[62] Garzoni transforms Tixier's lists of names and qualities into an

---

L'hospedale contains a section taken from Tixier's text. Garzoni does not use Tixier's *Officina* in chapters XVII ("Lunatics and Episodic Crazies"), XXII ("The Merry, Sweet, Facetious, and Loving"), XXVI ("The Obstinate, Like a Mule"), and XXVII ("The Hairless").

[59] "On Forgetfulness and Those Who are Deprived of Memory" and "On Folly and Those Who are Judged Insufficiently Wise." The first heading is under chapter VI, entitled "De artibus liberalibus ac manuariis, item de variis etiam artificibus." The second is part of chapter VII, entitled "De variis virtutibus ac viciis" (734–35; 1182). On the use of Tixier's index see Monica Calabritto, "The Subject of Madness: An Analysis of Ariosto's *Orlando Furioso* and Garzoni's *L'hospedale de' pazzi incurabili*" (Ph.D diss., City University of New York, 2001), 137–40 and Garzoni, *L'hospedale*, ed. Fiorato, 22–25.

[60] See the stories about Messalla Corvinus, the Thracians, Coroebus, and Calvisius Sabinus that Garzoni uses in the sixth discourse, "Of forgetful and demented fools."

[61] Garzoni uses one heading, "De furiosis ac maniacis" (*titulus* IIII, 504 ff.), for the discourses on the "melancholic and savage men" and on the "mischievous madmen" ("pazzi dispettosi o da tarocco"). Another heading, entitled "de gula, voracitate ac vinolentia" (*titulus* VII, 1260) is adopted for the discourse on the drunk madmen. Finally, the heading "De iis qui sibi variis modis mortem consciverunt aut se aliis occidendos commiserunt" (*titulus* IIII, 561) was adopted for the discourse on the desperate madmen and for that on the eccentric and extreme madmen.

[62] Ortensio Lando translated long sections of Tixier's *Officina* under the title of *Sette libri di cathaloghi a varie cose appartenenti, non solo antiche, ma anche moderne* (Ferrara,

explanatory catalogue of madness in its various forms and manifestations. The many portions of Tixier's encyclopedia displayed in Garzoni's text serve multiple purposes: in the first six *discorsi* they are used with the function of medical anecdotes, in contiguity with the ones taken from the medical treatises of Altomare and Fernel. In the other discourses, Tixier's short stories constituted a classificatory organization of madness in ancient times.

While Tixier's *Officina* stores knowledge concerning the gods, the animal world, the organization of time and its divisions, and humankind and the activities related to it, Giraldi's *De deis gentium* is an example of Renaissance onomastics and pagan mythography. It is divided according to sections dedicated to one god or goddess or groups of lesser divinities.[63] Giraldi's *De deis gentium* was widely read and influential: Natale Conti (*Mythologiae*, 1551) and Vincenzo Cartari (*Le immagini con la spositione de i Dei degli Antichi*, 1556) both relied on Giraldi's work.[64] Garzoni uses Giraldi's *De deis gentium* and *Vita Herculis*, a short work dedicated to the hero's life and deeds, in writing the prayers that are inserted at the end of each discourse dedicated to masculine madness. Each prayer to the god functions as an ex-voto, which the narrator offers on behalf of the patients for their healing. Thus the cure for masculine madness is metaphorical and depends on the action of an external agency, that is, a pagan divinity. As with Tixier, Garzoni conisiders Giraldi's text as a sort of dictionary, the content of which holds old and new elements together.[65]

Like Renaissance medical treatises and commentaries on Hippocrates and Galen's works, Renaissance encyclopedias had the task of organizing the knowledge transmitted by the ancients.[66] The main difference between the two genres consisted in their readership. While the medical treatise served an elite group of specialized people whose language long remained Latin, and collections of anecdotes and myths like Tixier's *Officina* and Giraldi's *De deis gentium* respectively addressed young students who were learning rhetoric and learned men interested

---

1552). Like Garzoni, Lando did not acknowledge his original source, but listed it as one among several others used in his work. For further analysis on the relationship between Lando and Tixier, see Cherchi, *Enciclopedismo*, 27 and 143–63, and idem, "L' *Officina* del Testore."

[63] Lilio Gregorio Giraldi, *De deis gentium* (Basel, 1548; facs. repr. New York: Garland, 1976).

[64] For an analysis of Giraldi's *De deis gentium*, and the relationship between this text and Conti's *Mythologiae* and Cartari's *Le imagini*, see Jean Seznec, *The Survival of the Pagan Gods*, trans. Barbara F. Sessions (New York: Harper Torchbooks, 1953), 229–43.

[65] For a brief analysis of the prayers in *L' Hospedale*, see Calabritto, "The Subject of Madness," 141–43.

[66] "Renaissance encyclopedias have the very practical function of organizing the whole of knowledge, which at the beginning of the sixteenth century is various, tumultuous, contradictory and unstable because of the humanistic discoveries of Classical literature and because of the scientific and geographical discoveries" (Cherchi, *Enciclopedismo*, 35).

in the rediscovery of pagan mythology in the Renaissance, Garzoni's *L'hospedale* addressed various categories of readers in the vernacular, including women.[67] His texts made available material previously limited only to those who could read Latin to a much larger public, and so did other intellectuals of the period, in the wake and rise of a flourishing market of printed books in Italian.

Gendered madness in and out of *L'hospedale*

While the language of sixteenth-century medical tradition contributed to gender certain types of madness, such as melancholy, *amor hereos*, and *furor uterinus*, the definition and the cure of madness in medical practice and within the hospitals tended to blur the distinctions between genders.[68] Both men and women were subject to melancholy, and the cure for both was based on the principle of expulsion and purgation of the organism. Social and moral deviance could be the reason for internment, while the medical categorization was secondary. In several Italian hospitals the most important thing was not curing the patients, but their internment and control within the space of the hospital.[69]

Individual admission to hospitals that treated patients perceived as mad depended also on the financial situation of the person and on the lesser or greater involvement of family members in his or her internment. Hospitals funded and financed by religious confraternities and groups accepted indigent people of both genders who were not considered dangerous to themselves or others, in order to take them out of the street and feed them. Other hospitals required a fee from their patients.[70]

---

[67] A female audience is the addressee of Garzoni's *Le vite delle donne illustri*.

[68] For an analysis of gendered melancholy and lovesickness, see Carol Thomas Neely, *Distracted Subjects: Madness and Gender in Shakespeare and Early Modern Culture* (Ithaca: Cornell University Press, 2004), 69–135.

[69] In the hospital of Santa Maria della Pietà in Rome the figure of the doctor was not very important in the admission of the patients, but it became essential at the moment of their release: see Bonfigli and Fedeli Bernardini, "Gli esordi," 49. Vittorio Biotti argues that in Florentine hospitals a more specific medical approach came to the fore only at the end of the sixteenth century: "Il folle nella società fiorentina e toscana del XVI e XVII sec. e la nascita di 'S. Dorotea de' Pazzarelli'," in *Follia, psichiatria e società: Istituzioni manicomiali, scienza psichiatrica e classi sociali nell' Italia moderna e contemporanea*, ed. Alberto de Bernardis (Milan: Angeli, 1982), 170–210, esp. 184.

[70] At the hospital of Santa Maria Della Pietà, people were admitted on a charitable basis when the institution first opened in 1548. However, a few decades later the patients had to pay to be admitted and their treatment varied according to the amount of money they could donate to the institution. See Bonfigli and Fedeli Bernardini, "Gli esordi," 46–48. In sixteenth-century Florence, a request from members of the family or from the community to the grand duke of Tuscany, rather than a medical examination, led

Once in the hospital, the patients were divided according to their gender but also according to their social status.[71] At the hospital of Santa Maria della Pietà, members of the confraternity and paid employees took care of the more affluent patients, while the less fortunate patients were located in separate wards according to gender, but they were treated regardless of the illness that affected them. These patients did not have individual cells, but lived together in communal spaces, except for the raging mad, who were located in a separate section of the hospital, probably in order not to create havoc among the other patients. Women and men were enclosed in their respective sections, even though occasionally they were allowed to take a stroll outside, like in Rome. However, most of the female patients—young women, raging maniacs—were progressively excluded from going outside, and mad women were usually forced to remain within the walls of the hospital for the rest of their lives.[72] For them, the cure was work rather than medical treatment.[73] Women were considered inherently deficient; their intellect and their will were weaker, while their passions were stronger. Whereas mad women's sexual appetite likened them to prostitutes, their forced enclosure and work conditions likened them to nuns.[74]

Unlike the complex vocabulary that university physicians adopted to define different categories of madness, the language used to define patients of both genders within the hospitals was very generic: they were "pazzi," "matti," "matti furiosi," or "melanconici." Medical knowledge was not as important as the community's perception in deciding the internment of mad individuals, regardless of

---

individuals of both genders to the incarceration in the prison of the Stinche. See Biotti, "Il folle," 182. For an overview of Florentine Renaissance hospitals see John Henderson, *The Renaissance Hospital: Healing the Body and Healing the Soul* (New Haven: Yale University Press, 2006).

[71] Like the hospital of Santa Maria della Pietà in Rome, many other Italian institutions had separate wards for men and for women, which were located in different parts of the building. For the organization structure of this hospital, see Bonfigli and Fedeli Bernardini, "Gli esordi," 2: 49.

[72] "The situation of women in the insane asylum is not very different from the condition of women in the other institutions: [they are] progressively enclosed, they are shown to the city with increasing caution, they work and will never leave the institution": Bonfigli and Fedeli Bernardini, "Gli esordi," 2: 51.

[73] At the hospital in Rome, while men at least for a certain period were kept inactive, women spun tow. See Franca Fedeli Bernardini, " 'Il vasto casamento della romana misericordia': Note per una storia delle istituzioni assistenziali nella Roma post-tridentina," in Bonfigli and Fedeli Bernardini, eds., *Fonti*, 2:273–78.

[74] Religious confraternities and the Catholic Church itself established many of these hospitals, structuring the spaces and organizing the activities of the institutions by borrowing elements from the structure of the convent and its life. For an overview of religious confraternities in sixteenth-century Italy, see Christopher Black, *Italian Confraternities in the Sixteenth Century* (Cambridge: Cambridge University Press, 1989).

their gender. In the hospital madness was assimilated to deviance, and the cure aimed at reestablishing order in the individual's behavior by enclosing the mad patient within the hospital and by enforcing social, religious, and moral conformity outside the hospital.

In *L'hospedale* Garzoni genders madness in two ways. He uses medical and encyclopedic language to define masculine madness and the metaphorical language of *impresa* to define feminine madness. He also creates a specific space for each gender from which he narrates the actions that madmen and madwomen perform within it. At the end of the second discourse on the "frenetic and delirious" Garzoni describes the entrance of the cell and the image of the divinity that is supposed to protect them:

> Their cell in this Hospital has for its insignia the figure of Minerva, because she is the goddess who has to protect this kind of madman. So prostrate on the ground, let us implore her help with this following prayer for the cure of these poor brainless, witless men. (p. 59)

The nature of the space where the madmen are secluded is brought to the reader's attention at the end of each discourse, when the narrator/guide addresses a prayer to the divinity who protects each category and whose *insegna* (an image or device) overlooks the entrance. In fact, the space of masculine madness remains vague and can be assimilated to the rhetorical locus of the memory theaters. The entrance of the cell and the image of the protecting divinity maintain a somewhat concrete dimension, but not the space where the madmen live. When the reader/audience "enters" into the cell, a polymorphous space of quotations, borrowings, and allusions from the medical and the commonplace tradition welcomes them. A myriad of fictional and historical characters from the past and from the present occupies each cell. Hercules, whom Garzoni locates in the cell of the "The Violent and Beastly: in Need of Ropes and Chains" (p. 157), shares the space with the mythical characters of Ajax, Athamas, and Pentheus, with Ariosto's Orlando, and with figures that probably belong to the local lore—a soldier from Brisighella, Santin da Villafranca, Marchione da Buffalora, and Domenicone da Guastalla. These characters are examples of a specific category of madness and are located in the space of rhetoric. Words become objects because they are likened to images, which transform the mnemonic process into a visual parade. This process of mnemonic visualization becomes particularly clear in the prayer to the protecting divinity at the end of each discourse. The "device" overlooking the entrance of the cell helps the author remember the identity of the god or goddess that he is invoking. The device is the visual element that triggers the etymological anamnesis of the plethora of names with which the author gives identity to the god or the goddess.

At the beginning of the section dedicated to mad women, Garzoni emphasizes the physical isolation in which every woman lives, alone, secluded in a cell.

Instead of the multitude of characters from mythical and historical periods that populate the cells of madmen, there is only one woman in each cell, and often she is described as naked. These women live in the contemporary period, and the only concession to a more distant past is shown in the names, reminiscent of the Roman period: Marina de' Volsci, the "matrona" Claudia Marcella, Marzia Cornelia, Flavia Drusilla, or Tarquinia Venerea, to name a few.

Garzoni further likens the readers of *L'hospedale* to spectators who gaze into the cells in the section dedicated to feminine madness by describing the space of the cell to the accomplice gaze of the audience and emphasizing the performative aspect of the text: each room is a stage, which the door frames and the *impresa* above the cell makes permanent.[75] Garzoni also introduces figures absent from the masculine section, such as the "Messere" or Superintendent who appears to be the guardian of the building, his family, and some servants, who usually interact with the madwomen in a hostile way.

At the beginning of the section on women, Garzoni brings to the reader's/audience's attention two elements that further distinguish madmen and mad women. The *imprese* that overlook the entrance of each cell and that attempt to describe with an image and a motto each woman's madness constitute the first element, while the nakedness of most of them constitutes the second element.[76] Both elements define women as controlled and contained: the *impresa* freezes their identity by assimilating each woman to a fixed, permanent image, while the baring of their bodies makes them prey to the public's inquisitive gaze. Even though Garzoni never brings the reader's attention to the naked body of the patients after his initial comment, he makes it an implicit feature of the women's appearance and a device through which he and the reader/audience contain feminine madness.[77] The *Messere* or Superintendent of the hospital exercises an explicit form of control and hostile containment in creating the twenty-eight *imprese* that he has placed over the entrance of each cell. The naked bodies of the mad women are transformed into the abstract bodies of the *impresa*, from which the *Messere*, obeying Paolo Giovio's precepts, has banned as much as possible the representation of human bodies and of physical attributes that could remind

---

[75] "But, please, go over a little further and look at that cell that has its door open, where she [...]"; "Oh, don't mind to talk with that woman dressed in gray [...]"; "Further down watch carefully that woman who is so very pensive and looks toward the walls [...]."

[76] In *L'hospedale* twenty-eight out of the twenty-nine categories of feminine madness are accompanied by *imprese*. Ostilia Mutinense, who exemplifies the last category of "devilish madness," does not have an *impresa*.

[77] For the relationship between feminine madness and the use of *impresa* see Monica Calabritto, "Garzoni's *L'hospedale de' pazzi incurabili* and the Ambiguous Relation between Word and Image in Sixteenth-Century *Impresa*," *Emblematica* 13 (2003): 97–130.

the reader of the women's nakedness.[78] The naked body of the female patient is tamed into a rhetorical "body" of knowledge, constituted by the image and the words of the motto in Latin, which comprise the *impresa*.

However, Garzoni's apparent control of the woman's madness through the *impresa* is belied by two factors. One factor is the tension existing between the narrative sections that describe the events that led each woman to the hospital or the actions that characterize her behavior in the institution, and the description of the *impresa* as a whole. The second factor is the tension between the description of the image and the motto within the *impresa*.[79] In Garzoni, the link between image and words is difficult to interpret, thus producing a sense of ambiguity in the reader that also depends on the nature of madness and on the gender represented in the section where the *imprese* appear.[80]

Garzoni was well acquainted with the theoretical debate going on in the second half of the sixteenth century in Italy on the nature and function of the *impresa*, which produced a plethora of treatises between 1555, the year of publication of Giovio's *Dialogo dell'imprese militari ed amorose*, and 1654, when Emanuele Tesauro's *Cannocchiale aristotelico* was published.[81] In *La Piazza di tutte le professioni del mondo* Garzoni dedicated a discourse to the "professors of *imprese* and emblems," in which he gave an overview of the main topics of discussion present in sixteenth-century treatises on *imprese* written by authors like Alessandro Farra, Francesco Caburacci, Girolamo Ruscelli, Paolo Giovio, and Scipione Bargagli.[82]

---

[78] See Paolo Giovio, *Dialogo del'imprese militari ed amorose*, ed. M. L. Doglio (Rome: Bulzoni, 1978), 37; Calabritto, "Garzoni's *L'hospedale*," 113.

[79] Calabritto, "Garzoni's *L'hospedale*," 102. Dorigen Caldwell argues that *imprese* "engender many different interpretations" and that, without the creator's or the bearer's explicit interpretation, "most *imprese* did not have fixed meanings": Dorigen Caldwell, "Studies in the Sixteenth-Century Italian *Impresa*," *Emblematica* 11 (2001): 1–257, here 229.

[80] Calabritto, "Garzoni's *L'hospedale*," 102.

[81] For studies on sixteenth-century Italian *imprese* see, at least, Robert Klein, "La théorie de l'expression figurée dans les traités italiens sur les *imprese*, 1555–1621," *Bibliothèque d'Humanisme et Renaissance* 19 (1957): 320–41; Mario Praz, *Studies in Seventeenth-Century Imagery*, 2 vols. (London: The Warburg Institute, 1939–1947); Armando Maggi, *Identità e impresa rinascimentale* (Ravenna: Longo, 1998); Dorigen Caldwell, *The Sixteenth-Century Impresa in Theory and Practice* (New York: AMS Press, 2004). For Garzoni's use of the theoretical discourse on *imprese*, see Calabritto, "Garzoni's *L'hospedale*," 115–20 and Caldwell, *The Sixteenth-Century Impresa*, 174–75.

[82] Tomaso Garzoni, *La piazza*, discorso XXVIII. Alessandro Farra, *Settenario dell'humana riduttione* (Venice: Christoforo Zanetti, 1571); Francesco Caburacci, *Trattato di M. Francesco Caburacci da Imola. Dove si dimostra il vero, et il novo modo di fare le Imprese, con un breve discorso in difesa dell'Orlando Furioso di M. Ludovico Ariosto* (Bologna: Giovanni Rossi, 1580); Girolamo Ruscelli, *Le imprese illustri* (Venice: Francesco

In *La Sinagoga*, Garzoni used Pierio Valeriano's treatise *Hieroglyphica*[83] and the tradition of hieroglyphs, which were very popular in Italy since the discovery of Horapollo's *Hieroglyphica* in the fifteenth century and were considered by some to be the prestigious forebears of the *impresa*.[84] For the *imprese* in *L'hospedale*, Garzoni used elements well known to an audience acquainted with the tradition of emblems, *imprese*, and hieroglyphs, but he changed their original meaning. In many *imprese* he manipulated the meaning of known images to fit a specific category of madness.[85]

According to several sixteenth-century experts, the link between words and images in the *impresa* is based on a metaphorical relationship.[86] Terms like comparison, similitude, proportion, convenience, and decorum were used to define the nature of the *impresa* and implied, at least in theory, a relationship of mutual influence between image and word. In practice, however, the balance between the two dimensions tends to privilege either the image or the motto. Each image possessed multiple and contrasting meanings, many of which were inherited

Rampazetto, 1566); Scipione Bargagli, *Dell'imprese* (Venice: Francesco de'Franceschi, [first ed. 1578] 1594).

[83] Pierio Bolzano Valeriano, *Hieroglyphica sive de sacris Aegyptiorum literis commentarii* (Basel: Isengrin, 1556).

[84] Horapollo lived during the Hellenistic period, probably in the fourth century B.C. He believed that Egyptian hieroglyphs were symbolic figures that expressed the wisdom of the ancients and their view of reality in a synthetic way, and relegated the analytical method, which was conveyed through words, to a subordinate place. Even though Horapollo's interpretation of the Egyptian hieroglyphs was wrong, it offered a convincing view to sixteenth-century intellectuals of the power of images and of the relationship between verbal and visual dimension. In 1419 the Florentine priest Cristoforo de' Buondelmonti bought the manuscript in the island of Andros and brought it to Italy. Aldo Manuzio printed the text in the original Greek in 1505 and Filippo Fasanini translated it into Latin in 1517. The edition that I consulted for the present study was printed in Paris in 1574. "The first to associate the *imprese* with Egyptian hieroglyphs appears to have been Mario Equicola, secretary to Isabella d'Este and Federico Gonzaga in his 1521 *Chronica di Mantova*": Caldwell, *The Sixteenth-Century Impresa*, 86, n. 132.

[85] Calabritto, "Garzoni's *L'hospedale*," 117. See pages 24–27 and our footnotes for the elaboration of known elements in Garzoni's *imprese*.

[86] Scipione Bargagli states that the "life" of *imprese* is a "similitude, or comparison" but also "metaphor and translation" of the their author or carrier, as does Emanuele Tesauro, who equates the notion of metaphor with that of proportion: Bargagli, *Dell'imprese*, 18–20; Emanuele Tesauro, *Idea delle perfette imprese*, ed. M. L. Doglio (Florence: Olschki, 1975), 55. See also Giulio Cesare Capaccio, *Delle imprese* (Naples: Gio. Giacomo Carlino, & Antonio Pace, 1592), 53, 75. Robert Klein argues that the link between the verbal and the visual dimension is based not on the assimilation of one element to the other, but on the notion of metaphor, of implicit comparison between the two terms: Klein, "La théorie de l'expression figurée," 339. See also Dorigen Caldwell, "Image in Imprese Literature," *Journal of the Warburg and Courtauld Institute* 63 (2000): 277–86.

from the hieroglyphic tradition. The motto kept the viewer from getting lost in a congeries of meanings and images by crystallizing the shifting dimension of the image into something permanent.[87] However, because of its polysemic nature, the image implied still other meanings that the viewer perceived and understood besides the one that the motto underlined.

In many treatises only a few of the *imprese* were visually represented on the page. The decision not to include all the *imprese* in the treatise might have derived from the fact that both author and reader knew the images described. Also, many texts were concerned with weighing the suitability of the visual dimension to a verbal description, making the text and its subject an example of "rhetorical oration."[88] In *L' hospedale*, Garzoni eliminates the visual dimension to rely completely on the verbal, descriptive dimension. Since there is no image to interpret, there are no multiple meanings to disentangle, and everything is explained through the words of the author.[89] However, several of the women seem to escape the interpretive cage that Garzoni gives them through the *imprese*. In the case of Domicilia Feronia (p. 194), for instance, an example of "ridiculous madness," Garzoni deprives the woman of her humanity by comparing her to a giraffe. Domicilia's madness is identified with her uncontrollable laughter, and her *impresa* represents an owl, " a ridiculous animal," with the motto "*Haec aliis et mihi alii*" (This [owl is a laughing matter] to others and the others [are a laughing matter] to me). Alciato considers the owl, an animal traditionally linked to Athena, goddess of wisdom, as the symbol of silent prudence, while Valeriano lists multiple meanings, from wisdom to victory, and from hypocrisy to Christ's humility.[90] If Domicilia's madness has reduced her to a giraffe, it does not completely imprison her in the frame of Garzoni's *impresa*. Women who make people laugh are dangerous, Garzoni seems to say, and the *impresa* helps the author distance himself and the audience from the madness of the patients. For Domicilia's laughter, Garzoni provides the fictional audience visiting the hospital and the reader with a scornful grin of superiority over her ridiculous and deviant nature.[91]

Garzoni further distinguishes feminine madness from masculine madness by portraying several female patients performing daily activities within the walls of the hospital. When describing the actions that madmen have performed before their internment and that seem to be the causes or the symptoms of the

---

[87] Scipione Bargagli compares the polysemic image to a palace left in the dark, made of many rooms and apartments. Only in one of these rooms one can find the "signore" of the building: Bargagli, *Dell'imprese*, 76.

[88] Calabritto, "Garzoni's *L'hospedale*," 118.

[89] Calabritto, "Garzoni's *L'hospedale*," 104.

[90] In the 1546 Latin edition of Alciato's *Emblemata* the owl is accompanied by the motto *prudens et infacundus*. See also Valeriano, *Hieroglyphica*, 146v.

[91] Calabritto, "Garzoni's *L'hospedale*," 108.

men's madness, Garzoni uses the commonplace tradition, but when he describes the actions performed by the mad women he seems to rely exclusively on the popular tradition contemporary to his own time.

Garzoni portrays women performing domestic activities within their own cell and other menial activities around the hospital.[92] The compulsory work to which women were subjected in some Italian hospitals, like that in Rome, might have influenced Garzoni's description, but the oddity with which these women perform activities like washing the laundry, sewing, spinning, and sweeping the floor stresses their inability to live in a domestic environment, where women were supposed to spend most of their life. Garzoni's women appear to transgress the equation work/cure more than submitting to it. Ultimately, it seems that in Garzoni's hospital there is no cure for the female patients. Unlike the prayer at the end of each discourse in which the narrator wishes for a recovery of the male patients, not even work seems to discipline and heal mad women.

Some women are also described as having contacts with sane persons who are not mad and work for the institution and with people coming from outside the hospital or with other inmates. Other women are described going in and out of their cell and are allowed visits by outsiders.[93] Giacoma di Panzipane, example

---

[92] Marina de' Volsci (p. 190-1), example of feeble-minded madness, has all the tools to sew, even though she prefers to nail flies and spiders with her needle. Orbilia of Beneventana (p. 191) and Tadia da Pozzuolo (p. 192), examples respectively of demented madness and of foolish madness, are supposed to spin, even though their lack of memory or wit keeps them from accomplishing the task. Orsolina of Capoana (p. 192), example of dumb madness, is ordered to sweep the floor or to wash the laundry in lye, even though her silly mind makes her do quite different things—cut her nails or blow air in the tub where the laundry is. Flavia Drusilla (p. 194), example of mischievous madness, is also described as washing the laundry at a nearby river; Andronica Rodiana (p. 195), example of feigned madness, sometimes goes into the barnyard and pretends to be a hen while she lays an egg, but when somebody approaches her to get the egg, she brandishes a club to keep him from getting closer.

[93] Quinzia Emilia (p. 197), who exemplifies joyful and jesting madness, has three men in her room with whom she converses about the fact that women are more mad than men and that nature had given them a weaker brain because she herself is a woman. Lavinia Etolia (p. 198), who exemplifies the category of extravagant madness, writes a grandiose letter in which she invites a woman of high rank and her servants to stay with her. Erminia of Bohemia (p. 198), a case of bizarre and whimsical madness, fights over chestnuts and dried apples with her fellow inmates for hours, and then she abandons the matter, as if she had never been interested in it. Calidonia da Eppi (p. 199) insults this and that woman, but when she comes back from the meal, her face is scratched and her hair is disheveled. Cecilia Venusia (p. 199), example of over–the–top madness, is described as being always surrounded by a circle of other inmates, because she "has introduced a climate of easy living here [in the hospital], which makes all the melancholic and wild moods go away." Lucilla da Camerino (p. 193), example of depraved madness, paints her naked body in black, and scares the women who belong to the guard's family out of

of beastly madness, is described as chained near her bed, probably because of her violent behavior towards other people.[94]

In some cases, Garzoni's iconic portrayal of some categories of madness glosses over the specific nature of each character's illness and focuses on qualities that are generically applied to large classes of individuals suffering from disturbances like melancholy, mania, and raging fury. However, other types of madness that allude to traditional classifications of insanity, such as natural dementia, love madness, and suicidal madness, do not present any iconic element.

While in the section dedicated to masculine madness Garzoni uses the medical tradition to define frenzy, melancholy, and loss of memory, in the discourse "On Madness in Women" he represents these categories through the description of the woman's behavior and sometimes through her physical aspect. Claudia Marcella (p. 190), example of frenzied and delirious madness, has hit her forehead against a stone, which caused her madness.[95] Physicians as well as uneducated people thought that hitting one's head could produce instant insanity or, at least, partial damage to one of the faculties contained in the brain.[96] Claudia Marcella has lost "her understanding and memory" and started "to rave and be delirious": now she thinks she is the Sibyl, and she sees herself in her chamber pot. Marzia Cornelia (p. 190), example of melancholic madness, who "stares at the ground, silent and melancholy, with her eyes lowered and all disheveled [...]" exemplifies the qualities that are usually connected to melancholy: fear of human society, desire for solitude, and an untidy aspect.

Even though drunken madness does not fit any specific category, physicians consider drunkenness a cause, a symptom, or even a cure for madness.[97] In

---

the kitchen where they are having their meal. Terenzia the Samnite (p. 197), example of clownish madness, summoned the guard's family into her cell to have them listen to a "very big belch, like a young sow," which she thought had to be honored by a crowd of people. Giacoma di Panzipane (p. 198) broke the chamber pot so hard on the head of a helper who had come to her cell to empty it that he was sick for days.

[94] Chaining or tying up was considered a normal procedure in this period. The patient was perceived as raging mad and therefore dangerous towards herself/himself and to others so that she/he was kept isolated from the rest of the community.

[95] The image and the motto of the *impresa* that accompany Claudia Marcella's (p. 190) madness are a bush of stinging nettles and the words "in puncto vulnus." There is no indication of any element that might help the reader make the connection between the image, the motto, and the case history. For an analysis of this *impresa* see Calabritto, "*L'hospedale*," 104.

[96] Antonio Benivieni narrates that a man hit on his head with a stone could not remember the alphabet; conversely, a madman who was hit on his forehead suddenly regained his wits: A. Benivieni, *De abditis nonnullis ac mirandis morborum et sanationum causis*, ed. G. Weber (Florence: Olschki, 1994), 195.

[97] Medical tradition believed that drunkenness produced effects similar to those that combusted melancholic humors had on one's brain. Some considered alcohol, and

the description of Teronia Elvezia (p. 191), Garzoni's representation of drunken madness possesses an overtly moralistic dimension, which he combines with a mocking tone directed towards the woman.[98]

Renaissance physicians considered conditions such as cretinism, dwarfism, and idiocy categories of madness.[99] Menega da Valtolina (p. 192), example of demented or stupid madness, has a goiter so big that she can throw it "behind her shoulders." Her physical handicap has an effect on her mental abilities.[100] Erotomania and suicidal madness are two other categories that are generally included in medical treatises but that Garzoni decides to treat as social and moral deviance. Her brothers and her parents confined Marzia Sempronia (p. 196), example of love madness, within the walls of the hospital, when they found out that she extracted a pound of her blood to send as a gift to the object of her desire, Quinzio Rutilio. Her family considered Marzia's behavior unacceptable and decided that the best remedy against this type of deviant behavior was to seclude the young woman in a hospital for mad people.[101] In the cell immediately after Marzia Sempronia's is Mansueta Britannia (p. 196), who, notwithstanding her name, represents desperate and suicidal madness, which was considered the final stage of melancholy and even love madness. Garzoni explains Mansueta's repeated attempts to commit suicide as the result of an overwhelming passion, which physicians could not cure, and the most insignificant elements can precipitate. Mansueta's attempted suicide because she had to give away a needle and

---

especially wine, a cure for melancholy and love madness, but others objected to the efficacy of this cure. See Mary Frances Wack, *Lovesickness in the Middle Ages: The Viaticum and Its Commentaries* (Philadelphia: University of Pennsylvania Press, 1990), for the position of several medieval doctors on the subject, and also Domenico Leone, *Ars medendi humanos* (Mantova: Giovanni Rossi, 1583), 99.

[98] In *La Sinagoga degli ignoranti* Garzoni accuses ignorant people of being gluttonous and drunkards. See in particular Garzoni, *Opere*, 513, where Garzoni creates a composite image of Bacchus made of the many qualities attributed to the god by the literary and emblematic tradition. The *impresa* for Teronia Elvezia's category of madness is a magpie holding a spoonful of soup in her mouth with the motto "Hinc silens, hinc loquax" ("Now silent, now talkative"). For an analysis of the *impresa* see Calabritto, "*L'hospedale*," 104.

[99] See Erik H.C. Midelfort, *A History of Madness in Sixteenth-Century Germany* (Stanford: Stanford University Press, 1999), 236–70.

[100] Menega's *impresa* is a bull with a hook in its nose and the motto "Quocumque rapior" (Lead me anywhere). For an analysis of the *impresa* see Calabritto, "*L'hospedale*," 105–6.

[101] "[…] thus, among rebukes and injuries she reduced herself to a desperate state of love madness, and when she reached it, her family, showing little charity, confined her to the place that you see." Marzia's *impresa* has a winged Cupid with a torch in his hands and the motto "desperata salus" ("Without hope of salvation"). For an analysis of the *impresa* see Calabritto, "*L'hospedale*," 111.

could not fix her pillow the way she wanted underlines the excessive nature of the woman's passion, especially for such petty motives, which makes her a completely irrational being.[102]

Analyzing how Garzoni perceives and represents some of the mad women engaged in daily activities and exemplifying in a more or less iconic way their form of madness does not imply that Garzoni is trying to portray a "real" hospital or to mirror the social reality of sixteenth-century Italian hospitals. Garzoni creates a space where rhetoric and the author's perception of madness as a social phenomenon meet and influence each other. While Garzoni privileges the rhetorical dimension of space in the section dedicated to masculine madness, he emphasizes its concrete dimension in the section dedicated to feminine madness, thus establishing a stronger connection between this part of his fictional hospital and the social reality of Italian hospitals. However, Garzoni's mad women are not historical individuals who can shed light on the way female patients were treated in hospitals for mad people in that period.

Garzoni constructs each example of feminine madness as if in relation with and in contrast to the corresponding discourse illustrating masculine madness. While men live in the rhetorical and abstract space of the medical and commonplace tradition, women are placed in the concrete space of the cell, where they live separate one from the other. While Garzoni describes the madmen performing no action within the walls of the hospital, he portrays the mad women performing domestic activities within and outside their cell and interacting with people considered "normal." However, women's reaction to work as a cure for their madness and their contact with the "sane" world—including the audience who watches them throughout the text—emphasizes their deviant status and their unpredictable behavior, rather than their growing adjustment to "normality." Garzoni implies a recovery for the madmen, through the prayer to a divinity at the end of each discourse. He offers no remedy for the women's madness and no hope that they leave the hospital. In the section dedicated to masculine madness Garzoni favors a narrative and analytical style, coupled with the exhortative mood of the final prayers. In the section dedicated to feminine madness he prefers a style that is more visual and iconic, in the sense suggested before, through the constant use of deictic adjectives that point out the space around each mad woman and the woman herself, and through an entire range of words that constantly bring to mind the visual dimension of which the woman is the object. He also describes some mad women by attributing to them certain qualities that render them the example of their category of madness, regardless of the individual

---

[102] The *impresa* of Mansueta Britannia has the trunk of a cypress with the motto "Semel mortua quiescam" ["Once dead I shall rest"]. The authorial control exercised over the mad woman through the *impresa*, that is, the correspondence between image and motto and the link with the bearer of the device, seems to lose its power against the concrete nature of the woman's behavior. See Calabritto, *"L'hospedale,"* 111.

nature of their disease. In the discourses dedicated to masculine madness the author invites the reader to perceive madness through the medical and the commonplace tradition. In the discourse on feminine madness he displays a range of various viewpoints from which the reader perceives the patients' abnormality and his/her own sanity. Garzoni puts aside the medical and the commonplace tradition and emphasizes popular anecdotes regarding the daily life of the female patients, which may allude to local contemporary lore.

Garzoni focuses his attention on vision, which is a means of control and containment, and which he expresses through the rhetorical device of the *impresa* created specifically for each woman. On the basis of Garzoni's stress on the visual dimension as a privileged expression of feminine madness, one can suggest that the author is more interested in containing and secluding feminine madness than masculine madness.

Conclusions

Garzoni's *L'hospedale* was composed when the ruling classes and the Catholic Church established norms to control and monitor the social and cultural activity of individuals within the community, norms which contributed to formulate what and who was considered "normal," acceptable, and appropriate. In sixteenth-century Italy the power tended to become centralized, giving more power to governmental institutions and to the aristocratic families that controlled them.

During and especially after the Council of Trent, the Church started to monitor the organizational structure of existing and of newly-created religious orders as a response to the climate of religious and spiritual reform that pervaded Italy since the end of the fifteenth century. The Church's goal was to create conformity within the religious institutions and within the community of believers. The pervasive diffusion of the printed text throughout Europe led the Church to exert a strict control over the material that individuals read and saw.

Garzoni operates a radical separation between sanity, which he equates with the notion of normality, and madness, which he assimilates to transgression and deviance. Garzoni's *hospedale* seems to fit perfectly Foucault's notion of confinement, with the exception that Garzoni writes about a fictional institution at the end of the sixteenth century, while Foucault writes about historical institutions that were established in the middle of the seventeenth century. Indeed, it is evident that Garzoni's treatment of madness and of mad individuals is more rigid and conservative than that which was used in contemporary hospitals in Italy. Garzoni's compartmentalization of madness depends on two main factors. The first is the generalized tendency to categorize and reduce reality to discrete fragments of knowledge. Consequently, if the mad individual, perceived as the "other" and the different, is reduced to an example to be catalogued, she or he is no longer dangerous. In fact, the phenomenon of compartmentalization is not limited to the subject of madness or to Garzoni's text but constitutes the prevalent attitude toward knowledge during this period. It is also connected in part to Church censorship, and the Church's desire to include knowledge and reality in a sort of encyclopedic, orderly universe. The second factor is constituted by Garzoni's treatment of gender, which consists in a radical separation between masculine and feminine madness, even though the classification in twenty-nine categories of insanity is identical. If it is true that Garzoni's intent is to contain madness, it seems that such a tendency is more marked in the section dedicated to feminine madness. Madwomen are "other" twice over: they are mad and they are women.

About this Translation

This present edition is based on the first edition of 1586. The copy used is contained in the Special Collections department at the Regenstein Library at the University of Chicago. We have aimed at an idiomatic English prose that nevertheless follows Garzoni's text closely. Some of Garzoni's idioms are obscure, and undoubtedly represent local, colloquial speech. Where we have not been able to track down an English equivalent, we have translated the idiom literally.

The notes for this edition include clarifications of obscure references—where clarification is possible—suggestions about the double-meanings and puns used liberally by Garzoni, and references to his primary sources. As noted above, Garzoni's "primary sources" were in most cases compilations of previously-published materials, in particular, John Ravisius Tixier's *Officina* and Giraldi's *De deis gentium*. It is often interesting to see how the original anecdote has been modified as it passes from the ancient writers, through Tixier, to Garzoni. We have noted the original references and their variations to faciliate further explorations of Garzoni's methods.

In the preparation of this edition, we have referred to three valuable modern transcriptions with notes: that of Paolo Cherchi in his collection of Garzoni's works (1993),[103] that of Adelin Charles Fiorato's dual Italian-French transcriptions (2001),[104] and that of Stefano Barelli (2004).[105] Notes from those three sources which contained information not verified from an inspection of the original source are followed by "Cherchi, [page number, note number]," "Fiorato, [note number]," or "Barelli, [page number, note number]."

---

[103] Garzoni, *Opere,* ed. Cherchi.
[104] Garzoni, *L'hospedale de' pazzi incurabili,* ed. Fiorato.
[105] Garzoni, *L'ospedale de' pazzi incurabili,* ed. Barelli.

The Hospital of Incurable Madness

L'Hospedale de' pazzi incurabili

Dedication

TO THE VERY MAGNIFICENT
SIGNOR BERNARDINO PATERNO[1]

ILLUSTRIOUS PHILOSOPHER
AND MOST EXCELLENT PHYSICIAN.

The illustrious name, and the rare fame, that—on speedy wings—has rapidly spread Your Excellency's boundless talents, and by now has penetrated into all parts of Italy; it has moved with such celerity that even within the bosom of my home town[2]—expanding like a brilliant flame—it revealed its light in such a way that, if these eyes of mine weren't more than greedy for the sight of its splendor, it would be solely out of envy that I would be able to pass in silence those things which your superabundant merits force me to make manifest because of my duty to the whole world. In addition, the report which I have received from many friends regarding the affection that Your Excellency has shown towards my writings—without my having ever deserved them—has represented your soul to my mind as so noble and generous that the more lowly and humble my works are, the more—because you elevate them with your judgment and intellect—you deserve that I, who have been made illustrious in the eyes of many, through your beneficence and favor, remain your servant, with perpetual ties of unwavering obligation, bound to honor you—with all possible effort—as my master.

So it should be no wonder, my most excellent signor, if, being urged on by the spur of gratitude—while at the same time moved by the vigor of your merits—I dexterously took the opportunity to enter the vast and spacious ocean of your praise, by dedicating to you this work of mine, the *Hospital of Madness*, which will be like the image of my love, and like an idea of your qualities because of the many places where the subject and the object correspond to each other. And what title, by Jove, would best befit the excellent profession of a very

---

[1] Bernardino Paterno (d. 1592) was one of the most famous Italian physicians of his time. Born in Salo, his father was a physician. He taught medicine at Pisa, Pavia, and Padua. See Jourdan, *Biographie médicale*, 6: 371. Paterno was the subject of a sonnet from "the unfortunate Tasso," a praise sonnet written about the time when the poet had been released from the Hospital of Santa Anna in Ferrara, where he had been kept by Duke Alfonso for seven years. The sonnet is "Superbo faro, ove le scienze e l'arti," addressed to Garzoni for his book *La Piazza universale*, in *Rime di T. Tasso*, ed. A. Solerti, 4 vols. (Bologna: Romagnoli-dall'Acqua, 1898–1902), 3: vi, number 1257; Fiorato, 11 and n. 14.

[2] "home town": Bagnacavallo, near Ravenna.

famous physician, than that of *Hospital of Incurable Madness*? It is only reasonable that a hospital be consecrated to the one who discharges patients by the thousands from the hospital, and that madmen should be consecrated to the one who enlightens schools and academies through his knowledge of his discipline, and that incurable infirmities should be consecrated to the one who frees infinite numbers of people from desperate illnesses through the Machaonian cure,[3] to use a saying by Battista Pio,[4] and like a new Asclepius, or a modern Apollo, gives life back to the dead, and preserves the living from death through his wholesome remedies. My excellent signor, let the ancients feel content to praise their Asclepiades of Prusa,[5] who rescued a man from his funeral—as they say—and saved him when he was considered dead; and that Critobulus,[6] who, with rare, praiseworthy ability, removed a deeply-embedded penetrating arrow from the eye of Philip of Macedonia, without disfiguring his face; and that Cheiron,[7] who gave sight back to Amyntor's son, Phoenix, who was completely blind; and many other truly accomplished and perfect personages in the medical sciences. But the modern age cannot stop boasting either, because Paterno has the soul of Galen, the spirit of Hippocrates,[8] and the guts of the father of this art, and can resurrect a Hippolytus,[9] bring back to life an Androgeos[10], and bring death itself back to life.

---

[3] "Machaonian cure": Machaon, son of Asclepius, was a famous surgeon of the Greeks during the Trojan War. Homer's epithet for him was "the incomparable healer": *Iliad*, 2. 732.

[4] "Pio": identified by Fiorato as Battista Pio (d. 1540), poet and philologue from Bologna. Fiorato, n. 5.

[5] "Asclepiades of Prusa in Bithynia": a famous physician, friend of Crassus. According to Pliny, he was "known most of all for having made a wager with fortune that he should not be deemed a physician if he were ever in any way ill himself, and he won his bet as he lost his life in extreme old age by falling down stairs": *Natural History*, 32. 37.

[6] "Critobulus": a Grecian physician. The anecdote is in Pliny, *Natural History*, 7. 37.

[7] "Cheiron," thought to be one of the wisest and most just of the Centaurs. He was distinguished for his knowledge of plants, medicine, and divination. He was a tutor of Aesculapius and Achilles. According to one version of the myth, Amyntor's mistress accused Phoenix of improper advances, so Amyntor put out his eyes. Cheiron restored his sight. Apollodorus, 3: 13, 8.

[8] "Hippocrates," of Cos, founder of the art of medicine.

[9] Asclepius restored Hippolytus to life. Son of Theseus and Hippolyte, he resisted his mother-in-law's (Phaedra) sexual advances. Out of revenge, Phaedra accused him of attempting to rob her of her chastity and his father cursed him and caused him to be torn to pieces by his horses. Propertius, 2.1.64, reports that Asclepius brought him back to life.

[10] Androgeos, or Androgeus, the son of Minos, was killed by jealous competitors after an athletic competition. According to Propertius (*Elegies*, 2.1.61-62) he was brought back to life by Aesclepius with Cretan herbs.

This, then, is the reason why I now dedicate this little work of mine to Your Excellency. And since I contrive to pray to the gods of the ancients to heal this sickly herd of madmen by means of several orations, I truly entreat you to strive to heal—as if you were a new Hippocrates—Democritus' insanity or, like a new Melampus of Preto,[11] that of the king of Argos, and that through your doctrine you may restore them and their lost wisdom, so that, in effect, the world may know that it has no father for its life and health other than the most famous and unique Paterno.[12]

It will do me no small honor in the world if there is an understanding that Your Excellency is the author, and I, the instrument of its sanity, providing that it will strive to obtain such a long break from its continued madness that it will be willing to accept the remedy, and become reconciled little by little to the diet of its madness.

Therefore enter the Hospital, Most Excellent Signor, and, at your own pace, see in what discomfort these madmen live and how much they need the visits of Your Excellency. In the meantime, I will wait outside, and will be a trumpet for your praise, hoping that my Hospital—being honored by the presence of your virtue—may soon reacquire its lost power, and be transformed into that castle of Atlante,[13] where people of all nations knew nothing but a content, happy, and tranquil life. With this I leave you, and I kiss the hands of Your Excellency.
Treviso February 25th 1586.
Your Excellency's humble servant
Thomaso Garzoni.

Sonnet By Policreti[14]
In Praise of the Author

A wiser, or more noble architect
The world never had; honor of our age;
That in a thousand ways challenges envy,

---

[11] Melampus, son of Amythaon, was thought by the ancients to have been the first mortal to have practiced medicine. He cured the women of Argos of their madness. Apollodorus, 2.2.

[12] Garzoni here plays on "Paterno" and "father" (*pater*).

[13] In Ariosto's *Orlando Furioso* cantos 2–4, Atlante tried to keep Ruggiero from joining the war by a series of ploys, the first being to entice him into her enchanted castle where he could be entertained by the worthy company of other knights and ladies.

[14] "Policriti": identified by Fiorato (n. 16) as Giuseppe Policriti, a writer from Treviso. See also Introduction, p. 5 and note 18.

And is more accomplished than Zeuxis and Pheidias.[15]
He, benign, sows for lazy intellects
The good path to their homes;
And if someone languishes in the shady cloister
He shows him his ailment, and accompanies him to bed.
And perhaps he discovers a deadly infirmity
In the one who believes himself healthier than all,
So that the insane populace may be derided.
This is the great compassion of one who strives
And does not strive in vain, to make known
The acts and deeds of madmen.

By the Same Poet on the World's Folly

Some measure steps with their feet;
Some speak Latin, without knowing nor understanding it;
Some contend within themselves along the way,
And some think they know something because they can throw stones.[16]
Some always laugh or always remain silent;
Some constantly expect to be saluted.
Some sing, dance, or offend people;
Some are amazed by everything.
Some are too insatiable, and some are too stingy;
Some let themselves be flattered by a lie
And some think they can equal Jupiter.
Of all these I would like to know, if you please,
Which is the most perfect and greatest folly?

---

[15] "Zeuxis and Pheidias": two of the most famous artists of Antiquity. Zeuxis (5th-4th c. B.C.) was known for the realism of his works. He is said to have died laughing at a portrait he had painted of a funny old woman. Pheidias (490–430 B.C.) was the greatest sculptor of antiquity.

[16] "throw stones," probably, "the simplest of acts."

Author's Prologue to the Spectators

The obvious vanity, the clear foolishness, the explicit madness of some miserable and unfortunate ones; with their heads bloated with haughtiness and the backs of their heads lighter than an oak-gall,[1] more void of sense than cockles at the waning of the moon; nevertheless, excessively presumptuous about themselves because they see that Fortune, that friend of buffoons (since, according to the Philosopher,[2] where there is a paucity of intelligence, there is where she hurries with the greatest enthusiasm) uplifts them to such a height that, like that squash immortalized by Ariosto, they crash to the ground in an exceedingly short period of time:[3] this is the irresistible reason why I, being in such a state of amazement and astonishment at so much madness, and after writing my *Theater of Minds*,[4] have decided to build this great *Hospital*, where their glorious madness can be seen, written in capital letters, in a separate ward, depicted by me with such a beautiful and masterful perspective that the other madmen will make a circle around them and, as the Kings of Madmen, they will receive a flood of applause from everyone, so that while the pot boils, the smoke which they enjoy so much may ascend along the Way of the Beret with ever-increasing power.[5]

This does not mean that the general madness of the world does not move me to address it as much as do its individual types, but these have so much power that I, in sympathy with the entire human race, have built a separate cell for each

---

[1] "*pan Cucco.*" Luigi Ferri, *Vocabulario ferrrarese italiano*, has *pan Cuch*. Garzoni explains later, in the oration to Hercules (Discourse 29), that it is "a fruit of extreme lightness." Garzoni may have also had in mind a play on "pan Cucco," with the added meaning of "universal cuckoo" or "grand kook."

[2] Aristotle discusses the relationship between wisdom and Fortune in *Eudemian Ethics*, 8: 2. 1–20.

[3] Ariosto, *Satire* 8 (179–81). A pear tree overgrown by a squash vine chides the squash for being so presumptious to believe that its vine would hold it up. The parable is told in Ariosto's letter in which he rejects any interest in high offices.

[4] Garzoni, *Il Theatro de' vari e diversi cervelli mondani*, "The Theater of the World's Various and Sundry Mind." First published in Venice (G.B. Somascho, 1583), it is a description of 55 different types of personalities or temperaments. In Garzoni, *Opere*. No English translation is available.

[5] In other words, the vain pleasure of so much attention—represented as rising smoke—goes straight to—and out the top of—their heads.

one where they can all be comfortable and repose with the greatest of ease. And with respect to this, you will see how pious the author of this structure has been, for not only has he built this edifice to meet the needs of so many sick people and those with impoverished brains, but he has also sought—with brilliant inventiveness—to commend every single one of them to some god under whose protection they may be assisted, or, better yet, helped with and protected from their madness—to the extent that this is possible.

So he will fervently pray to Minerva to help frenetic or delirious madmen; to Jupiter, the Hospitable One, the melancholic or unsociable; to Apollo, the loafers or careless; to the god Abstemius, the drunkards; to Charon, the forgetful or demented; to the god Sentinius, the dumbwits, who are as good as lost and dead; to the Ox of Egypt, the dull, bloated, gross-witted, and those who are fooled; to the Samian Ewe, the retarded and air-heads; to the goddess Bubona, the jerks and giddy; to the god Fatuellus, the clumsy and vain; to the goddess Themis, the perverts; to Nemesis, the spiteful and tarot types; to the god Risius, the laughable; to Juno, the vainglorious; to Mercury, the fakers and burlesque types; to Hecate, the lunatics and episodic crazies; to Cupid, those madly in love; to the goddess Venilia, the desperate; to Vulcan, the heteroclytes, the odd, brain-damaged, or incurably crazed; to Fabulanus, the buffoons; to Bacchus, the merry, sweet, facetious, and loving; to Tisiphone, the bizarre and frenzied; to Mars, the raging and beastly, those who should be tied up or, even better, put in chains; to Hercules, the extravagant and extremely senseless; to Rhadamanthus, the brazen ones; to Volutina, the excessive or the triple-refined; to Hippona, those unbridled like a horse; to inexorable Minos, those stubborn as mules; and, finally, to infernal Pluto, madmen deserving of the gallows a thousand times over, or the diabolical.

In the meantime, the author will pray to the Penates,[6] that they may take good care of this household of the world's madmen; and to the Tutelaries[7] that they will take on the guardianship of this new hospital; and to the goddess Ops, that, with appropriate remedies, she will assist so many who are infirm and devoid of all sense; and to the goddess Meditrina, that she will medicate them well; and to the god Aesculapius, that, with the miraculous hellebore,[8] he will purge them thoroughly; and to the goddess Sospita, that she will heal them completely; and to the god Janus,[9] that he will let anyone pass through the door of this hospital in order to see the misery of these unlucky and unfortunate ones. And most

---

[6] "Penates": the household gods of Rome.

[7] "Tutelaries": gods whose function is to protect the city and its inhabitants.

[8] "hellebore": name given to several species of the genera Veratrum and Helleborus, used as treatment for madness, epilepsy, and paralysis, thought to act via its powerful purgative properties: Barelli, ed., *L'Ospedale*, 11, n. 11.

[9] Ops, goddess of abundance; Meditrina, goddess of healing; Aesculapius, god of medicine; Sospita, or Juno, goddess of redemption; Janus, god who looks both backwards and forwards and hence rules over the opening and closing of doors.

importantly, that on that day when one celebrates All Fools' Day, as the Romans did, it is the wish of this author that they throw open the doors so that one can see the Bacchanals of the Maenads,[10] a thing most odd and enjoyable to see.

With this invention, therefore, he wishes to blunt the temerity of those modern Thersiteses who consider themselves Ajaxes;[11] of those pigmies who hold themselves up as Alcides; of those tarot-idiots[12] who deem themselves Nestors; of those country crickets who act so much like parrots; of those perched cuckoos who make fun of the whole world; of those shell-less slugs who raise their antennae for nothing; of those pine-woods gadflies who fly off from cow-dung; of those jump-toys properly fitted with lead in their feet and with heads lighter than straw: because as they walk through this hospital, they will see that Silliness is their mother, Buffoonery their sister, Melonheadedness their life's companion. Between them and madness, a logical equivalence is created, a physical relationship, and an identity good enough for a follower of Scotus.[13] These are the ones who placed the whim into the head of the author to author this new structure where the honored spectators can take great solace and enjoyment from gazing on the foolish *prosopopeia*[14] of these savage geese. They will take no small delight and pleasure from these odd, never-before-heard-of follies which, in this place, will be discovered in those that, acting like Cato[15] among the masses, will ultimately reveal themselves to be Masters of the Grasshoppers or Doctor Graziano or Merlin Cocais,[16] which is what they really are.

---

[10] The Maenads are associates of Bacchus or Dionysus, known for their wild, licentious festivities and dances. See D. Brumble, *Classical Myths and Legends in the Middle Ages and Renaissance* (Westport, CT: Greenwood Press, 1998), 48–52.

[11] Thersites, famous for his cowardice, is juxtaposed to Ajax, the valiant warrior; pigmies are juxtaposed to Alcides (one of Hercules' names); and idiots are juxtaposed to Nestor, the quintessential wise man.

[12] "tarot-like," or *tarocco*, suggesting the notion that those who invoke Tarot cards are idiots. Garzoni's Counter-Reformation sensibilities are evident here, where tarot card readers are scorned. Also, more generally, a madman without any redeeming qualities.

[13] A follower of Duns Scotus (ca. 1266–1308). Scotus, also called 'Doctor Subtilis,' was known for the intricacies of his philosophical arguments, not all of them comprehensible.

[14] "*prosopopeia*": the rhetorical device whereby a concept is personified.

[15] "Cato": probably Cato of Utica, known for his sagacity, to whom the *Distichs* (a school text) were ascribed. Another Cato, M. Porcius Cato, was a Roman patrician famous for his haughty pride in his family, even though his family had never been recognized with honor by the Roman magistrates. Hence, another example of presumptuous folly.

[16] Dr. Graziano, stock character of the Commedia dell'Arte, usually portrayed as a pompous, but ignorant scientist. Garzoni will refer to him repeatedly in *The Hospital*. Merlin Cocai is the pseudonym of Teofilo Folengo (1496–1544), author of a famous satirical poem, *Baldus*, written in macaronic Latin. "Merlin Cocai" may be translated as "Merlin of Baby Chicks." For Teofilo Folengo, see also Introduction, p. 3 and note.

Therefore, those who want to be entertained will pay at least a *venti*,[17] because this is no two-bit comedy nor some trivial slapstick routine by Gradella[18] which is put on in the marketplace as an antipasto for Magaleppan plums.[19]

The first thing which will be shown will be a monster with many heads, which will amaze everyone with its deformity: neither the Hydra, nor Medusa, nor Python[20] were so horrible and frightening as this one. And then, one by one, we will see this palace of the magician Alcina, room by room, full of people whose brains have been enchanted and transformed, through a bestial metamorphosis, into stupid and irrational people.[21] There, between laughter and amazement, everyone will be pleased to have spent their twenty bucks in this way, departing from the author well-satisfied. He will also show you — with new magic — the castle of Atlante,[22] full of madmen, and he will try to lead you to safety with Logistilla,[23] placing in your hand Angelica's ring,[24] which will enable you to uncover the madness of others and thereby appear to be that much wiser.[25] So stand back while he unleashes the monster. And keep your eyes posted if you want to be amazed from the very start.

---

[17] "*venti*": twenty soldi, a rather considerable sum.

[18] Gradella, usually "Gradellino," stock character of the Commedia dell'Arte: Cherchi, 253, n. 16.

[19] "Magaleppan plums," originally "balle di Macaleppo." A play on "*balle*," meaning both the fruit of this plum-like tree and "plums" as foolish folk. Cherchi (254, n. 17), and Barelli (14, n. 28) provide alternative suggestions. Magaleppa or macaleppa refers to a tree of the plum family.

[20] The three most horrible and vicious monsters of mythology.

[21] Ariosto, *Orlando Furioso cantos*, 6–7. Alcina, a sorceress, transforms her visitors into trees and animals.

[22] *Orlando Furioso*, 2:38. The magician Atlante built an enchanted castle in the Pyrenees in order to entertain his protégé, Roger, and make the Paladins victims of their own illusions and hallucinations. See also, p. 38, note 12.

[23] *Orlando Furioso*, 10. Logistilla was the half-sister of Alcina, and, as her name implies, she represented the force of reason which was able to dominate the passions. She saves Astolfo and Roger from the charms of Alcina, and therefore ends by destroying the kingdom.

[24] In *Orlando Furioso*, Angelica's ring magically makes her and others invisible. Garzoni invokes her ring to make his spectators invisible as they journey through the Hospital. See Orlando Furioso, VII, 65-71 and VIII, 1-2.

[25] Garzoni has limited expectations that this journey will actually make the spectators wiser; only that they will "appear to be" wiser.

The First Discourse:
Universal Madness

Since I have shouldered the burden of presenting to the world the amazing varieties of Folly—she, with a countenance more deformed than Cadmus' serpent,[1] uglier than the Chimera,[2] more venomous than the dragon of the Hesperides,[3] more noxious than Corebus' monster,[4] more terrible than the Minotaur of Theseus,[5] more horrible-looking than three-headed Geryon[6]—who has descended into our world in order to vomit forth the flames of her poison, like Hercules' wild beast,[7] in order to injure and inflict pain on us all, regardless of one's particular situation, it is essential that I describe her in such a way that, simply by virtue of your view of her, all will be overwhelmed and terrified, and the whole world will be prepared to affirm that the Harpies[8] did not stink so much, that

---

[1] The dragon, an offspring of Ares, god of war, guarded a spring to which Cadmus sent his men for water. The dragon was subsequentially killed by Cadmus.

[2] The Chimera is variously described, but in one popular version had the body of a lion, the head of a dog, another head of a goat on its back, and the rear of a dragon. It was said to breathe flames. See Brumble, *Myths*, 54–55.

[3] Argus, the monster of one hundred eyes. The dragon assisted the Hesperides in guarding the golden apple which Ge had given to Hera on her wedding to Zeus. See Brumble, *Myths*, 35.

[4] This monster, Poene, had been sent into the country of the Argives by Apollo to destroy them but was killed by the youth Corebus.

[5] Usually depicted with a human body and a bull's head. See Brumble, *Myths*, 223–24.

[6] Geryon, king of Hesperia, had three heads and three bodies. One of the Labors of Hercules was to steal Geryon's oxen. For all the labors see Brumble, *Myths*, 156–59.

[7] The Lernean Hydra, a monster with nine heads—the middle one immortal. Hercules killed it as another of his Labors.

[8] Monstrous birds that looked like women. They earned the epithet "foul-smelling" with their defecating on Aeneas' dining table. Fiorato (n. 45) suggests that Garzoni's long list of monsters suggests that he viewed fools as having a type of bestial monstrosity. See Brumble, *Myths*, 147–48.

Hercules' bull was not so full of pestilence,[9] nor that the sea monster, Hesione,[10] was not so damnable as she.

Once she enters the domain of the brain, she obfuscates the imagination, perverts thought, alienates the mind, corrupts reason, and so impedes a man that he cannot understand, choose, speak, nor do anything right, but instead, with troubled fantasies, he is like a vacillating spirit, sick reasoning, a brain in agony, a head as vacuous as a dried-up watermelon; he wanders aimlessly, like a millhorse, around a thousand sillinesses, as pitiable as he is ridiculous.

But the worst thing that is born from her is this: that by continuously fuelling pain in the brain, she makes one so stupid and out of one's mind that the crazier he becomes, the wiser he thinks he is. At that point when he considers himself to be another Mercury, he is really a Corydon or a Menalcas[11] among the masses. This happens because, as Hippocrates states in his *Aphorisms:*

Quibus ita mens aegrotat ij dolorem non sentiunt.

Those with infirm minds feel no grief. [12]

Therefore Folly is she who, when spread and disseminated throughout every province and country in the world, unbearably afflicts mortals, and she holds vast numbers of people subject to her tyrannical empire, so that what is said in Ecclesiastes is only too true:

Stultorum infinitus est numerus.

The number of fools is infinite.[13]

---

[9] The raging bull which Hercules caught on Crete and rode over the sea to Mycenae. See Brumble, *Myths*, 158.

[10] Garzoni takes this reference from Apollodorus, 1. 208, where Hercules, in full armor, leaped into the jaws of the sea-monster Hesione and for three days hacked at it with his sword. When he emerged, he had lost all of his hair. "Hesione" is also the name of the daughter of Laomedon, king of Troy. Because he refused to pay Apollo and Poseidon for their work in building the walls of Troy, Laomedon was obliged to give up Hesione to a sea monster sent by Poseidon against the reign. Hercules agreed to save her: Apollodorus, 2: 207–9.

[11] The two shepherds of Virgil's *Bucolics* (Eclogue 2). Cherchi notes that they are not as stupid as Garzoni's contrasting of them with Mercury would suggest (Cherchi, 254, n. 12) but Garzoni uses them here, and elsewhere, as paragons of simple-mindedness.

[12] Hippocrates, *Aphorisms* 2, 6. Cherchi (p. 254, note 13) points out that the original text is slightly different.

[13] Ecclesiastes 1:15.

And just as Harpagus[14] did with his own son's brain—not just impiously, but villainously—so she grinds her monstrous teeth against this one and that one, seeking to satisfy the greedy longings of the human brain. She does not spare kings, has no respect for emperors, holds no captain in esteem, does not consider the learned, pays no attention to the rich, has no fear of nobles, and has no regard that may stop her, striking a hailstorm of blows, this way and that, at all mortal offspring.

Behold the ancient grip that this beast has held over the world, so that the people of Agathyrses, near Syrtes—the first of all madmen—as a sign of their obvious folly, walked around naked, with their bodies painted in various colors like the spotted leopard.[15] So Virgil wrote, in Book Four of the *Aeneid*,

Cretesque Dryopesque fremunt pictique Agathyrsi

Cretans, Dryopës and painted Agathyrsians raise a shout.[16]

The Andabates, portraits of true madness, were inclined to fight their wars blindfolded.[17] The Arcadians—utter madmen—thought that they were older than the moon. Because of this Seneca, in his *Hippolytus*, said:

Aut te stellifero dispiciens polo
Sidus post veteres arcades editum.[18]

---

[14] "Harpagus" in Herodotus, *Histories*, 1:117–20. King Astyages gave his daughter's son to Harpagus to kill, but Harpagus couldn't comply, out of pity. As punishment, Astyages arranged for Harpagus to eat his own son. After dinner, Harpagus was presented with his son's head, hands and feet. Astyages then asked Harpagus if he knew what he had eaten. He replied, "Yea, I know, and all that the King does is pleasing to me." Rather than Garzoni's categorization, it would seem that Harpagus could be termed a heartless madman, and Astyages the cruel one. Garzoni seems to have relied on Tixier's brief note (*Officina*, 3:33) rather than Herodotus. Harpagus is briefly noted by Ovid, *Ibis*, 545–546: "Like the young son of Harpagus mayst thou recall the example of Thyestes, and, carved in pieces, enter thy father's bowels."

[15] These examples, from the Agathyrsians to the Tonemphians, are taken from Tixier, *Officina* 7. 48. Fiorato (n. 54) points out that Garzoni repeats Tixier's error of describing the Agathyrsians as living in Syrtes when, in fact, they were from the region of the Black Sea.

[16] Virgil, *Aeneid*, 4:145–146. The Agathyrsians tattooed their bodies to indicate rank and also dyed their hair a dark blue. They were also said to have kept their wives communally so that all would feel related to one another.

[17] The Andabates were gladiators who fought with their visors completely closed, blocking their vision.

[18] Seneca, *Phaedra*, 785–786.

... the star, created after the ancient Arcadians,
Watches you from the stellar pole.

The Himantopodes, truly fatuous, zigzagged along the ground on their hands and feet, like snakes.[19] The Mendesians—lacking judgement in all things—bestowed the greatest possible honors on the labors of their goatherds.[20]

According to Herodotus, the Psyllians—buffoons of the fourth degree—fought in armed bands against the south wind because it blew against them.[21]

The Ptoenphae, their brains veritably crippled, elected a dog as their king, and according to the way it turned, they inferred which commands they were to obey.[22]

But who does not see how much folly holds sway among men, especially when learned men, who should be wiser than the rest, prove themselves to be more foolish, asserting things that baby blackbirds would not believe. The baby magpies of Valcamonica would hardly utter the nonsense that they speak.[23] Isn't Pliny's tale of Philetas of Cos a fine one? He was a compiler of elegies, whose body was so light and subtle that it was necessary to fasten lead weights to his feet so that a puff of breeze would not blow him away.[24] And what about those other two, written about by Ausonius and Pontanus?[25] Caeneus and Tiresias[26] changed

---

[19] Himantopodes were mythical people of Ethiopia.

[20] Mendesians were inhabitants of the Nile delta.

[21] The Psyllians were ancient people of Libya. Herodotus reports, "The force of the south wind dried up [their] water-tanks, and all their country, lying within the region of the Syrtis, was waterless. Taking counsel together they marched southward ... and when they came into the sandy desert, a strong south wind buried them": *Histories* 4: 173.

[22] The Ptoenphae were an Ethiopian tribe. Pliny, *Natural Histories*, 6.35.

[23] Valcamonica, in the Italian Alps, north of Bergamo and Brescia, was known at that time for the clumsiness of its inhabitants: Fiorato, n. 246.

[24] Philetas, a grammarian and Greek poet. All of the examples from Philetas to Lymira are taken from Tixier, *Officina* 7 (1049). The Philetas anecdote is also in Aelianus, *Historia varia*, trans. Diane Ostrom Johnson (Lewiston: Mellen Press, 1997), 9.14 (198). Claudius Aelianus was a Roman polygraph of the second century, author of a celebrated collection of historical and literary anecdotes, the *Historiae variae*. Fiorato, n. 71.

[25] Ausonius, poet and Latin rhetorician from Bordeaux where he lived most of his life (ca. 310–395). He was a professor of rhetoric, tutor of Gratian (Gratianus Augustus) and Saint Paulinus of Nola, and finally a councilor. His familiar poetry or descriptives (*Domestica*, *Mosella*) were widely appreciated. Giovanni Pontano was an illustrious poet, humanist, and statesman from Naples (1426–1503) who was in the service of the Aragon family of Naples. His scientific, moral, and literary works exerted a significant influence on the culture of the kingdom of Naples and on humanism at the end of the fifteenth century.

[26] Ausonius, "Epigrams on Various Matters": 76 in *Ausonius*, 2:199. Tixier, *Officina* 7:52 (1049). For Caeneus, see also Virgil, *Aeneid* 6.448–449. For Tiresias, see Ovid, *Metamorphoses* 3.316–340.

their form from male to female, just as a potter turns a drinking vessel into a pot while the clay is still moist and supple.

Another tale from Pliny is equally delightful. On the lake at Tarquinia,[27] there used to be two groves of trees that were carried about, sometimes in a triangular or square configuration, and other times circular.[28] Nor does this other one taste like fennel seed:[29] that the herb called *achaemenis*,[30] when thrown among enemy troops, has the power to make them turn their backs and run away in spite of themselves.

Licinius Mutianus[31] is not impolite when he reports that he saw a woman in Argos called Arestusa who married a man, and on her wedding day she turned into a man, growing a beard and male genitals. Later, as he reports, she took a wife, since she had been transformed into a man.

Similarly, that other tale presented by Celio[32] does not reek of chamomile. A certain Marino, who resembled a man above and a horse below, died three times and, miraculously, was three times raised from the dead.

The tale of Aelianus[33] is no less weighty than the others: Ptolemy Philadelphus had a deer trained so that it clearly understood his master when he spoke Greek.[34]

Another of Pliny's tales is no less fantastic. In Lymira, in a fountain in Lycia dedicated to Apollo, the fishes, called three times by the sound of a bagpipe, obey the sound and surface without delay.[35]

---

[27] Probably Lake Vico, near Tarquinia (Latium): Fiorato, n. 67.

[28] Tixier, *Officina*, 7.52 (1049).

[29] A saying meaning "Nor is this other one tasteless."

[30] "achaemenis": Tixier, *Officina*, 1051 and Pliny, *NH* 26.9 (7: 279).

[31] Licinius Mutianus, Roman politician, member of the Triumvirate in the second century A.D.: Tixier, *Officina* 7.52 (1049); Pliny, *Natural Histories* 7.3.

[32] Celio Rodigino, or Ludovico Ricchieri from Rovigno (1469–1525), humanist known for his *Ancient Lectures*, one of Garzoni's most frequently cited sources. This work was published six times in the sixteenth century. The first edition was *Lectiones antiquarum libri XVI* (Venetiis: Aldi et Andreae soceri, 1516). Fiorato believes that Garzoni probably used the edition in thirty volumes published in Basel by Frobenius, 1566. The anecdote about Marino can be found in 5:45 of the 1566 edition. However, it can also be found in Garzoni's principal source, Tixier, *Officina* 7 (1049) where the author cites Celio.

[33] The anecdote is not to be found in *Historiae variae*, but is in Tixier, *Officina* 5.52 (1052).

[34] Ptolemy Philadelphus was king of Egypt in the third century B.C.: Tixier, *Officina* 5.52 (1051).

[35] Pliny says "At Myra in Lycia at the fountain of Apollo whom they call Surius, the fish, summoned three times on a pipe, come to give their augury. If they tear the pieces of meat thrown to them, this is good for the client, if they wave it away with their tails, it is bad": Pliny, *Natural History* 32: 8.

But Pedro Mejia[36] tells a story derived from other sources that is really unbelievable. A certain king, Cipus, had intently watched two bulls fighting one day. Afterwards, he went to sleep with the image of them deeply impressed into his mind only to awaken later to discover that he had sprouted bull's horns from his head.[37] This man may have been a follower of the philosopher Protagoras who—foolish ninny that he was—was so impudent that he stated that whatever seems to be the case is, in fact, true. Plato devoted some effort to scolding this madman who deserved the gallows a thousand times over, saying that if this proposition were true, then it seemed to him that Protagoras had uttered sheer nonsense, which, according to the same principle, was certainly true.[38]

But anyone who tries to fully describe all the crazy stories that learned men have foisted upon the world, and to mention all the crazy actions that the men of this world have done, would have taken on a burden that would weary Atlas himself—not to mention the feeble wit and weak memory of an ordinary writer like me.

May it suffice to righteously affirm, with the Teacher, that:

Vidi cuncta, quae fiunt sub sole, & ecce universa vanitas, & afflictio spiritus.[39]

I have perused all things done under the sun, and behold, all is vanity and affliction of the mind.

The Egyptians, too, certainly were very foolish and vain by worshiping onions, leeks, and the heads of garlic for their gods, as Juvenal asserts in his fifteenth Satire.[40] The Babylonians also lacked reason, since they worshiped the god Belus by offering him enough meat to eat that they could have fed a thousand people with it.[41] And the Romans could well be numbered among those triple-refined

---

[36] Pedro Mejìa (or Mexía), humanist and Andalusian historian (1497–1552), author of a vast compilation, *Silva de varia lección* (1540). He was the historiographer for Charles V: Fiorato, n. 72. See also, Introduction, p. 10 and note 31.

[37] Cipus, a Roman praetor, was also said to have sprouted his horns as he was leaving the city. The *haruspices* said that if he returned to the city, he would be crowned king. Since he didn't want to be king, he imposed exile on himself: Ovid, *Metamorphoses*, 15. 565 and Pliny, *Natural History*, 11.37, 45.

[38] Plato, *Theaetetus*, 160D.

[39] "The Teacher," the author of Ecclesiastes. The line is a paraphrase of Ecclesiastes 1:14.

[40] Juvenal, *Satires*, 15.9. Garzoni may also have had in mind the note on "garlic and onions" in Pliny, *Natural History*, 19:101. The example is also found in Tixier, *Officina* 7.48 (1007).

[41] Belus was the son of Libya and Poseidon, who ravished her. Libya was the daughter of Epaphus, son of Io and Zeus. Belus was also called "the Egyptian Zeus," and was worshipped in several Middle Eastern countries.

jokers[42] by offering divine sacrifices to a slut like Flora,[43] and by worshiping Stercutius[44] as a god, making him, no less undeservedly than shamefully, preside over latrines and shit.

But why am I narrating the follies of the ancients when our own time is the image of madness itself, or, rather, a veritable closetful of all of the world's vanities committed by men? When were the bizarre notions of the alchemists ever in greater estimation than they are now, so that many great people humiliate themselves by going to the furnaces and blowing the bellows onto the crucible in order to become members of the sect of Geber and Morienus,[45] all of them more crazed than a horse? When were Ramon's[46] crazy cabalistic teachings more frantically sought after—he who, with his most imperfect art, intended to make asses dance like Barbary horses and make them capable of galloping at full speed even though, by nature, they are only able to trot? When have there been so many copies of handbooks and almanacs full of lies? At Rialto[47] one can even find the ridiculous prognostications of a man who consumed one hundred eggs in a morning to avoid entering the madhouse. Yet this miserable creature could not avoid the malignant influence of the stars and planets and his own infelicitous constellation, for he was forced to enter into The Hospital for Incurable Madness as a two-bit astrologer, because that is how much his compositions sell for in the marketplace. When have there walked on this planet so many quacks and mountebanks who claim to be physicians with degrees from the University of Bologna, when, in fact, they turn out to be nothing more than pig-castrators

---

[42] "matte da tre cotte," literally thrice-cooked fools. "Tre cotte" is used in reference to highly purified sugar, hence "triple-refined," an extremely high-quality fool.

[43] Flora, Roman goddess of flowers and spring, was worshipped by a cult centered on the temple of Castor and Pollux. In an attempt to discredit her, later Christian writers viewed her as a courtesan, with a large number of lovers.

[44] Stercutius, one of Saturn's many epithets, was also the name of the Roman god of excrement and manure, presiding over the fertilization of the fields.

[45] Geber, or Djahir, an Arabic alchemist of the eighth and ninth centuries. Some consider him the founder of alchemy. Morienus, a Roman alchemist, probably legendary, who lived in a monastery in the Orient. To him are attributed celebrated texts such as *De re metallica, De metallorum transmutatione,* and *De compositione alchemiae.* A modern English translation of one of his works is available: Morienus, *A Testament of Alchemy being the Revelation of Morienus, ancient Adept and Hermit of Jerusalem to Khalid ibn Yazid ibn Mu'Awiyya, King of the Arabs of the Divine Secrets of the Magisterium and Accomplishment of the Alchemical Art,* ed. and trans. L. Stavenhagen (Hanover, NH: University Press of New England, 1974). These two alchemists exerted a significant influence on science in the Middle Ages: Fiorato, n. 81.

[46] Ramon Lull (1233–1315), celebrated theologian and Catalan missionary, known during the Counter-Reformation for his occultism: Fiorato, n. 82. See introduction, page 10.

[47] Rialto: the great Venetian marketplace which surrounds the famous Rialto bridge.

from Norsia[48] who would just as soon sell pork gristle instead of vials of salve for the itch? When was there such an abundance of seekers after new secret formulae? Even in Bergamo there was a man who bragged of knowing the secret for converting the Turks, and he would have sold it to a physician friend of mine for a piece of forty if he wanted it. It was such an important thing that if Fioravanti of Bologna[49] had known about it, he would have despaired that he had not included it in his *Medical Fancies* under the title *Fioravanti's Divine and Angelic Elixir.*

When were there so many uncivil dunces as there are today, who, not with the understanding of Archimedes but with that of a *cabalao* or swindler,[50] build an attic latrine in place of a dovecote and a snake-puddle in place of a fish-pond?

To conclude, all the world is full of madness from top to bottom, and one man pecks his brain into one form,[51] another into a different form. One goes crazy for earthly glory, considering himself a veritable Triumphal Arch, when in fact he is worth less than a cobbler. Another soars high with four *cuius* that he learned by heart[52] as if he were an archduke of the ancient world—Greek as well as Latin. Another laces his breeches holding their pointed laces tight because he can boast he has ten *scudi* in his control, ones that he could hardly amass after fasting for twenty years. Another acts like the king of Cappadocia,[53] like a rooster, sword drawn, because he sees himself promoted to some wretched hangman's position, as if everyone didn't know that putting a responsibility in the hands of a clumsy oaf is like giving a donkey a harp to play.[54] Another melts into broth and jelly just for having a retinue of four ragamuffins around him, like a Phrandone[55]

---

[48] Norsia, or Norcia. Village in the Umbrian Apennines whose inhabitants were known as great butchers and, at least in Garzoni's time, also skillful charlatans: Fiorato, n. 86

[49] Leonardo Fioravanti (1518–1588), celebrated medical charlatan and follower of Paracelsus, author of various works, who attributed his powers to his great "secret," the Elixir Fioravanti. The Elixir was still in use in the nineteenth century as an antidote to arsenic poisoning. See P. Camporesi, *Camminare il mondo: Vita e avventure di Leonardo Fioravanti medico del Cinquecento* (Milan: Garzanti, 1997). See also, Chapter 5, "Leonardo Firovanti, vendor of secrets," *in* William Eamon, *Science and the Secrets of Nature: Books of Secrets in Medieval and Early Modern Culture* (Princeton: Princeton University Press, 1994).

[50] The terms also echo "interpreter of the Cabala," one of Garzoni's *bêtes noires*.

[51] "pecks his brain." The idiom suggests thinking about trivial matters; wool-gathering.

[52] Here Garzoni makes fun of the sticklers for grammar.

[53] King of Cappadocia, a play on words, meaning both that and also a rooster: Cherchi, 260, n. 40.

[54] Compare Erasmus, *Adagia*, 1.4.35 *"asinus ad lyram,"* "A donkey listening to a lyre": 31: 344.

[55] Phrandone: possibly a corruption of Pantalone, the Commedia dell'Arte mask. His frequent adversary, Dr. Graziano, the pompous, ignorant scientist, was fond of annoying Pantalone by garbling his name, for example, Piantalimone, Petulon, and Pultrunzon. See K.M. Lea, *Italian Popular Comedy*, 2 vols. (Oxford: Clarendon Press, 1939), 1:18.

of buffoons in the midst of Sorian monkeys.⁵⁶ Another really acts like Signor Cappocchia⁵⁷ and the Know-it-All of Letters because he feels as important as the king-pin at the bowling green, as if the game would end without the pin feeling the ball on its head.

And thus at the table, everyone discards both the good and the better, without considering what the wise man said, *Vanitas vanitatum, & omnia vanitas*,⁵⁸ that is, "Vanity of vanities, all is vanity." But because we will know our subject better in general if we discuss the particular types, let us move little by little to the particular types of madmen, so that we may achieve that complete and perfect knowledge of madness which we seek.

---

⁵⁶ Garzoni also continues to play with the word "*sori*," now referring to "Sorian monkeys," with one meaning being "vacuous" or "air-headed" monkeys, the other, monkeys from Soria in North Africa. "Soria" sometimes refers to "Syria," but this meaning seems less likely here.

⁵⁷ "Cappocchia": a silly person.

⁵⁸ Ecclesiastes 1:2.

THE SECOND DISCOURSE:
THE FRENETIC OR DELIRIOUS

The general opinion of all learned physicians about that condition which we call Frenzy—and especially of Galen in the first of his *Prorrhetics*[1]—is this: Frenzy is the proper term for that affection or inner distress which, associated with high fever as its symptom, brings ongoing dementia in the brain of the patient.[2] This distress, as Aëtius wrote on the authority of Poseidonius,[3] is an inflammation of the membranes of the brain that induces a delirium and a very grave assault to the mind. Therefore those who experience this unpleasant and uncanny distress are termed frenetic and delirious. But Trallianus,[4] that excellent physician, in the thirteenth chapter of his first book, is of the opinion that frenzy is an

---

[1] This first paragraph, with all the weightiness of scientific citations, is taken, almost verbatim, from the first paragraph of Chapter 7, "*De phrenetide*," of Donato Altomare's *De medendis humani corporis malis* (Naples, 1553), 34. Donato Antonio Altomare (ca. 1520–1556) was a Neapolitan physician and follower of Galen. He specialized in pharmacology and was the author of an *Ars medica* (Naples, 1553 and Lyon, 1565) which went through six editions during Garzoni's lifetime. He is Garzoni's principal source of medical information. He also wrote a *Medicinae praxis in qua iuxta...* (1597): Fiorato, nn. 99 and 104. See also, Introduction, p. 14ff.

[2] In this section, Garzoni describes inflammatory disorders of the brain, such as syphilis, which, at certain points in the course of the illness, are associated with hyperexcitable behaviors or "frenzy" as well as signs of delirium. Garzoni does not make the distinction clearly delineated in modern medicine between *delirium*, an ordinarily reversible lowering of consciousness associated with a wide variety of medical conditions, and *dementia*, a chronic, usually progressive disorder of the brain associated with evidences of irreversible neuropathology.

[3] Aëtius of Amida, Greek physician (sixth century A.D.), the author of a vast compilation of Galen's works in six volumes, *Tetrabiblion*. Poseidonius, Greek philosopher and historian of the second century B.C., born in Syria. He is said by some to have continued the *Universal History* of Polybius, although others question this attribution. See Fiorato, n. 101.

[4] Alexander of Tralles, Greek physician of the fifth century A.D. Author of a therapeutics in twelve books frequently used during the Middle Ages. He was termed "the greatest Greek physician after Galen" according to J.D. Berger and J. Billen, *Dictionnaire des auteurs grecs et latins*: Fiorato, n. 102.

inflammation of either the brain or its membranes. And Paulus Medicus,[5] in the sixth chapter of his third book, proffers his opinion in this way: Frenzy is an inflammation of the membranes of the brain, though sometimes the brain appears to be inflamed, while at other times it presents a certain heat, which is different from that which we call natural heat.

Furthermore, Galen, in the second book of his *On the Causes of Symptoms*,[6] clearly maintains that both the brain and its membranes are the seat of the distress. Most physicians agree with him, and in particular, among modern physicians, we find Altomare, in the sixth chapter of his *Medicinal Method*.[7]

But physicians distinguish between frenzy and delirium, although both of them are associated with a fever, because delirium — as John Fernelius Ambianus,[3] in the fifth book of his medical works, has written — is sometimes caused by bile and sometimes by an effusion of thin blood into the brain, and sometimes by other causes. But frenzy is always caused by that inflammation of the brain mentioned above. In addition, most of the time delirium is a symptom of fever or some other more serious malady. However, fever is not a symptom, but is the cause of frenzy. Delirium occurs fairly often, but frenzy is very rare. Frenzy is a far more violent illness than delirium.

Because I don't wish to speak about madness the way physicians do, but rather according to the plain talk of the people, I have subsumed both frenetic and delirious madness under one heading, because when one speaks *bus* and *bas*[9] about something, we ordinarily say that he is speaking like a frenetic or delirious madman, since that person is undergoing the same experience as those who are properly afflicted by delirium or frenzy.

---

[5] "Paulus Medicus," or Paul of Aegina, "the last of the classical Greek physicians," seventh century A.D. He travelled widely and practiced surgery and obstetrics in Alexandria. His work *De re medica libri septem* was published in Basel in 1532 and 1546 and was republished twenty times during the sixteenth century: Fiorato, n. 103. An English translation was made by Francis Adams: Paulus Aegineta, *The Seven Books*, 3 vols. (London: The Sydenham Society, 1847).

[6] *De causis symptomatum*, in C.G. Kühn, *The Works of Galen*, 7:147–204.

[7] Altomare, *Medicinae praxis: in qua iuxta Galeni doctrinam miro ordine traditur ars curandi humani corporis mala* (Venice: Sessa, 1597).

[8] John Fernelius Ambianus, or Jean Fernel of Amiens (1497–1558), called "the Modern Galen," one of the most famous physicians of his time. He taught in Paris for the greater part of his career: Fiorato, n. 105. See also, Introduction, p. 12 and note 43.

[9] A "*bus* and a *bas*," a poke at pompous classicists who argue over arcane matters of Latin grammar, such as which ending should be used, *-bus* or *-bas*. Barelli (27, n. 10) suggests that the phrase here means to be delirious. Cherchi has suggested as an additional possibility that it means "sound without sense": "In bus e in bas," *Lingua Nostra* 29 (1968): 108.

The Frenetic or Delirious

So I call frenetic and delirious madmen the ones who, in a sort of realization[10] of true delirium and true frenzy, are constantly out of their minds, are inconsistent in their speech, and get so convoluted that the Sphinx would have difficulties disentangling their ideas, and Oedipus would sweat to understand the sense of their words, because their speech shows great facility, but their phantasms ride on the back of Pegasus, wandering first this way, then that, without direction.[11]

Regarding this type of madness, two examples may suffice for the learned man. A certain Sparsus is mentioned in Seneca's *Epistles* as showing these conditions:[12] among scholars he talked like a madman; among madmen he held forth like a scholar, so that in both situations his delirium was evident to all. The second example comes from the much-esteemed author Celio—in the ninth book of his *Ancient Lectures*[13]—where he describes a certain decrepit woman—and mind you, delirium seems to be proper to old age rather than to any other age—called Acus, who, seeing her face in a mirror, deformed by old age, went crazy because of the great pain that that view caused her. In her madness, she spoke to her face in the mirror, laughed, and would confabulate with it. Sometimes she would threaten her image; sometimes she would make promises to it; sometimes she flattered it; sometimes, becoming more frenetic, she would get angry with it; sometimes as happy as an Alcina, and other times like another Gabrina, full of resentment and spite. [14]

But among the common folk, we can add the example of that old cuckoo, Talpino from Bergamo—who was under no obligation to think normally for more than a quarter-hour plus one minute at a time—who traveled from Bergamo to Venice for a hearing before the Council of Forty to appeal a verdict decided against him regarding a certain house on which he had a claim. As he stood before them, he suddenly skipped from talking about the house to the well, and maintained that he would at least lay claim to the house's well. He insisted with such obstinacy that the Signors, laughing, offered to make him the proprietor not just of the well, but of the whole sea. So he gave up his claim on the well, and carried the news back to Bergamo that the Councillors had made him Lord of the Sea as well as of the *Bucentoro*.[15] But when he returned to his former state

---

[10] "realization," the mind's capacity to imitate or reproduce a state of mind.

[11] *Sphinx...Oedipus*. Oedipus solved the riddle of the Sphinx.

[12] Seneca the Elder, *Controversiae*, 1.7.15 (1:171). The story is also in Tixier, *Officina* 2:60, "On Frenzy and Mania."

[13] "Celio." Although Garzoni cites Celio for this story, it is not in the *Ancient Lectures*. Tixier, *Officina* 2:60 (215).

[14] One of only two examples of a woman in this part of the Hospital. For Alcina, the sorcerer of Ariosto's *Orlando Furioso*, see p. 44, note 21. Gabrina is another old crone from the same source.

[15] Bucentoro, the Doge's ceremonial barge used in Venice's grand naval festivals, particularly the "marriage to the sea," a ceremony in which a gold ring was thrown from

of mind, he had another issue with the Council: that, as Admiral of the Seas, it seemed to him a great shame that he had a great a quantity of salt water for his ships to sail on but had no fresh well water to supply to them. So with that, some of the Signors, noting his mental leaps, and, for the amusement of the assembly, had a document made up for him, signed in charcoal[16] and sealed with a mark good for branding horses, in which they declared that they had presented to him for his use all the waters of the rivers of Serio, Oglio, Brenta, Sile, Piave, Tagliamento, Gravallone, Adige, and that part of the Po which flows within their dominion.[17] But in the end, the fool concluded that he didn't want so much water but just his house. Otherwise, he would burn Bergamo to its very foundations, together with its chapel.[18]

No minor case of delirium is the one described of Santino of Tripalda, who got the idea of going to the University of Padua at the age of sixty-four. Arriving at an inn near the school, he had them point out to him the most famous physician teaching at the University at that time. He entered the lecture hall at the hour of the class, along with the other students, and while the professor was lecturing on matters of the brain,[19] he began to shake his head as vigorously as he could. Finally, unable to contain himself any longer, and—in the presence of all the students who, at first, because of the old guy's nice appearance, did not understand in which foot he was lame[20]—he cried out that he wanted to maintain this conclusion: that the dumb oxen of Tripalda had more brains than all the professors and students in Padua. With that, the scholars flocked around the newly-revealed madman and, with much laughter, had him immediately take the lecturer's chair, desiring to hear what *bons mots* this new arch-professor had to offer. So he hopped up to the lectern, but while they expected one thing, he gave them something different. He started talking about how to defeat simultaneously both the Turks and the Sufis. Then he jumped into a discourse on the Grace of St. Paul,[21] just as charlatans do. Then, he was quickly on to telling about how he had escaped from the hands of the Turks. Finally, he arrived at this proposal: that although he had come to Padua in order to become a doctor, and because he

---

the Bucentoro into the sea as a sign of marital domination of Venice over the sea.

[16] Erasmus explains (*Adagia*, 1.5.54) (2:430): "*Creta notare, carbone notare,*" or "to mark with chalk for approval; to mark with coal to condemn."

[17] All rivers in the vicinity of Venice which were under its control at the time.

[18] The chapel of Colleoni, condottiere of Venice in the fifteenth century, situated off the main square in Bergamo; built by Giovanni Antonio Amadeo between 1472 and 1476. Fiorato, n. 117.

[19] "matters of the brain," a pun on *materia*, meaning both "matters" and "foolishness."

[20] "in which foot he was lame," i.e., "what kind of fool he was."

[21] "Grace of St. Paul" was soil taken from the grotto of San Paolo in Malta, thought to be miraculous, which Umbrian charlatans—"the Ceretani"—sold as a cure for snakebite. See Paolo Cherchi, "La grazia di San Paolo," *Lingua Nostra* 30 (1969): 120.

had heard that the scholars of Padua study a thousand subjects, he wished to do a public lecture in this University on the *Orlando Furioso*, without salary, providing they would then be satisfied that his were the very best lectures. All consented for fun, and all shouted with one voice, "Long live Santino of Tripalda," since during his presentation he had revealed his identity. Descending from the lectern, he turned to all of those assembled and said, "Classmates, let everyone perform his part, and I will leave the lectern empty. *In sequenti lectione*, I will return to Tripalda having been made a doctor by your graces."

Therefore, those who have a brain like Santino of Tripalda and Talpino of Bergamo are to be included among those fools whom common folks term frenetic or delirious. Their cell in this Hospital has for its insignia the figure of Minerva,[22] because she is the goddess who has to protect this kind of madmen. So, prostrate on the ground, let us implore her help with this following prayer for the cure of these poor brainless, witless men.

A Prayer to the Goddess Minerva on Behalf of Frenetic and Delirious Fools

To you, O Tritonia, virgin, worthily adorned by a thousand other epithets, as Tritonia of Itonia, of Lyndia, of Nedusia,[23] of Ionia, of Scillutia, of Alcides, of Sciras, of Alea, of Filetis, Polias, Glaucopis, the Attean Virgin, called Pallas by the Greeks (because, with a spear in your hand, you are considered the goddess of arms) and called Minerva by the Romans (because you rightly advise those who are in need of counsel), I affectionately address these, my humble prayers. And if you are — as all men consider you — the goddess of wisdom, born from Jupiter's brain, with reason called Operaria (because all sage operations proceed via your assistance),[24] called Nerine (which means potent, because your mind is constant and strong in all your deliberations), called by your name, Tritonia, preceded by the name Dedala by everyone (which means ingenious, because you are the mother, mistress, and lady of human ingenuity), I pray to you, who are all mind and reason, take care of these souls who are forsaken by wit, abandoned by reason, who resort to you through me. You know that whatever they utter is said

---

[22] Minerva, goddess of wisdom, ironically invoked to look over the witless. However, another of her epithets is *Frenatrix Minerva*: Lilio Gregorio Giraldi, *De deis gentium, libri sive syntagmata XVII [. . .]* (Lyons, 1565), 347. For Giraldi, see Introduction, p. 13, note 43 and p. 20.

[23] Garzoni often alters the spelling of these epithets, perhaps to create a pun, although what the pun might be is unclear. For example, Giraldi, *De deis gentium*, has Nedusia, not Medusea as in Garzoni.

[24] She was also the goddess of artisans and of work.

with *crassa minerva*,[25] being in such a frenetic and delirious state that their case is commonly considered hopeless.

Therefore, relieve them of this mental delirium, heal this insanity, treat this frenzy, so that with their understanding recovered, their wits reacquired, their brains returned home, they may praise you, Goddess, principle, source, and cause of understanding and generator of mind. And now I say no more to you, most wise Goddess, for "a sow does not lecture Minerva,"[26] since you are the one who is able enough to teach the whole world, who holds the key to science, art, and all fields of knowledge and all of our understanding.

If you give salvation to these miserable wretches in your temple, a gourd will be consecrated to you. It shall hang at your feet as a sign of your having given intelligence to these fools who, like the gourd, were empty inside.

Rest in peace, and save those who need your help.

---

[25] "*Crassa Minerva*," in Manuzio, *Adagia* (63) and Erasmus, *Adagia*, 1.1.37 (31:85–86), number 37: inelegant or crude knowledge.

[26] "*sus Minervam*," or "a sow teaches Minerva": Erasmus, *Adagia*, 1.1.40 (31: 88–90). The adage refers to a fool who tries to teach a wise man. Also in Manuzio, *Adagia* (65), Garzoni's likely source.

The Third Discourse:
The Melancholic and Savage[1]

The most renowned physicians, both ancient and modern, join in this fundamental conclusion: that melancholy should be considered a sort of delirium that is not associated with fever, which is caused by nothing but an excess of melancholic humors which have occupied the seat of the mind. In fact, it is common to all melancholics that their brains are diseased, either essentially or by consensus, as Altomare[2] states in the seventh chapter of his *Medicinal Arts*. This is also Galen's opinion in the third book of his *On the Diseases and Symptoms of the Parts of the Body*[3] and of Hippocrates in the sixth book of his *On Common Disorders*, and of Paulus Medicus in the fortieth chapter of his third book,[4] and of John Fernelius Ambianus, in his treatise *On Various Diseases and Symptoms*, where he writes these very words: "Melancholy is an alienation of the mind, and those who are affected by it either speak or do absurd things, or things that are are very far from reasonableness or thoughtfulness. And all of these things they do with dread and sadness." Hippocrates considers these two signs—dread and sadness—as certain and infallible signs of melancholy.

But Donato Antonio Altomare—on the authority of Galen, in his second book, *On the Causes of Symptoms*, and Aëtius, in his special chapter *On Melancholy*,[5] and Alexander of Tralles, in the seventeenth chapter of his first book—proves that melancholic men have only their imaginative faculty affected, not their cognitive function or their memory, since they tend to be deceived by things that they see—which falls under faulty imagination, not the other two functions.

---

[1] In this section, Garzoni vacillates between using "melancholia," the scientific word, and "maninconia," the lay term.

[2] See p. 5, note 1 and Introduction, 14 ff. This reference is to *De medendis*, Chapter 7, "De melancholia," 42–50: Cherchi, 266, n. 1. Altomare notes two types of melancholy: one in which the brain itself is diseased, i.e., "essentially," and the other, in which the brain's disease originates outside the brain, and becomes disordered "by consensus" or in response to these outside influences.

[3] *De locis affectis*, in Kühn, *Works of Galen*, 8: 177–93.

[4] Paul the Physician, or Paulus Aegineta. See 55–56 n. 5 above.

[5] *De melancholia ex Galeno, Rufo, Posidonio et Marcello coll. Aetii Libellus*, in Kühn, *Works of Galen*, 19: 699 ff.

Similarly, all authorities agree that there are many different types of melancholic madness, which will become apparent during the course of this present work.

Among the various effects of this dementia, they describe these: melancholics have very little courage and valor; they are filled with sadness and fear without understanding its cause; they weep excessively; they wish to be alone; they hate being with other people; they abhor diversions and pleasures for a while and then, later—as Theodorus Priscianus,[6] says, in the second book of his *Medical Matters*—they regret having despised them, and then try to rejoin them. They long for death, and sometimes act to accomplish it. All of these effects are not always seen in the same subject, but sometimes create torment individually, and sometimes together. Therefore, we may find innumerable types of melancholic madmen, because the excess of humors[7] affects different people differently, causing greater or crazier effects in one person than another.

Galen, among others, in the third book of his *On the Affected Parts*, describes a man who, imagining that he had become a complete crock-pot, gave way to everyone he met, in order not to smash into them and hurt himself. And Altomare, in his treatise *Treatment of Diseases of the Human Body*, mentions two others: one, hearing a rooster crowing and beating its wings, also flapped his arms and imitated the bird's crowing and flapping. The other one feared that Atlas—whom the poets say holds up Mount Olympus—might become tired of holding this huge weight and might throw it down and he would be crushed under the mountain. So he was unable to stand up straight and had to continually shrink back, as if that massif were always about to fall on his head.[8]

Celio, in the twenty-sixth chapter of his ninth book, lists a man named Pisander among this sort of madmen. Thinking that he had died, he became wondrously afraid of running into his own soul, which he considered to be a mortal enemy of his body, and he was determined not to have anything to do with it, since it had treated him so badly and was so unfaithful in leaving him.[9]

But what is there to say of Nicoletto of Gattia, who, suffering from this indisposition of the brain, one day got the idea that he had turned into the wick of an oil lamp, so he wanted everyone to blow on him, from the front, from the back, and from the sides, fearing that he would burn out until he disappeared?

---

[6] Theodorus Priscianus, Greek physician of the fourth century A.D., who may have been associated with the court at Constantinople. He wrote a work on simple remedies, *Rerum medicarum libri quatuor* (Strasbourg, 1532).

[7] "Humors": here, black bile, the humor associated with depression and melancholy.

[8] This unfortunate melancholic may also have identified with the Atlas of the adage, *"Atlas coelum,"* or "Atlas held up the sky," said of one who gets themselves entangled in great and grievous matters, thus seeking out trouble for themselves: Erasmus, *Adagia*, 1.1.67 (31:110–12).

[9] For the episode of Pisander, see Garzoni, *Teatro*, Discourse 51. Although Garzoni cites Celio, this episode is found in Tixier, *Officina* 2.60 (215).

No less savage is the salty humor of this type, which afflicted Toniolo of Marostica, who, having been persuaded by his fantasies that he had turned into the heel of a shoe, went all the way to Vicenza with his ass to the ground and his feet in his hands, fearing that some cobbler along the way might accidentally tack him to his heels or soles.

No less gross, I believe, is that notion that came into the head of Bertazzuolo of Nuvolara. His wit having become seriously nebulous,[10] one day thought that he had been turned into a Chioggian watermelon, so he bumped his head against first this man's nose, then that man's, crying out that no one should buy him because it was not yet August.[11]

I will end the follies of these miserable sorts with the ridiculous example of Petruccio of Prato, who had taken to believing that he had turned into a mustard seed and threw himself hands and feet into a mustard grinder which a spice-merchant had outside his shop. So he caused eight or ten ducats' damage for the poor merchant, who could never have imagined such a thing.

Physicians include in this sort of melancholy a type of insanity which the Greeks call "lycanthropy" and the Romans call *insania lupina* or "wolf madness," which, according to Altomare,[12] causes men to go out of their houses on February nights, and, like a wolf, to wander among the gravestones howling, and pulling out the bones of the dead, dragging them in the streets, causing great fear and trembling in all who encounter them. And our author affirms that melancholic people like this have pale faces, dry and sunken eyes, and weak vision, and they don't shed a single tear. Their tongues are dry; they are extremely thirsty, and have an abnormally small amount of saliva. He also affirms having seen two men who were greatly troubled and oppressed by this type of malady.

On this point, Fornaretto of Lugo[13] is a notable example, who, suffering from this madness in his imagination and cognition—because all authors do not agree on memory—he went one night into the Jewish cemetery where an old Jew, over eighty years old, had recently been buried. The Jew had been sick from dropsy for more than six years. Fornaretto lifted the body onto his shoulders and took it to the piazza in front of the castle, and there he began playing with it as if it were a ball, crying, "Fault!" or "Serve!" or "Hit it!" or "Play ball!" Little by little he awoke the entire neigborhood, and the rumor went from person to person, through all of the Jewish households, that this man had disinterred Master Simone (for that was the dead Jew's name), and he created a wonderful Synagogue

---

[10] Garzoni makes a pun on *Nuvolara*, the town, and *nebulous*, cloudlike.
[11] And hence, he was not yet ripe.
[12] *De medendis*, Chap. 9, "*De lupina insania*." Also in Aëtius, *Libellus*, "*morbo lupino*," in Kühn, *Works of Galen*, 19: 719.
[13] Lugo: town about 2 miles west of Bagnacavallo, Garzoni's birthplace.

of Mirth[14] in their presence, seeing that the fool had taken an arm-bone to use as a bat in his ball games and the body, full of disgusting liquid, for a ball. And with every blow, the soupy mixture spewed out. It took two weeks for the community just to quell the stench. Even the stingier types preferred to pay one *carlino*—it would have been too painful not to have the piazza cleaned up—rather than to breathe in the perfume of Master Simone, which was no joking matter.

To this tribe belong melancholic and wild madmen. They have a cell in the hospital that is very much like the grotto of the Cumean Sibyl.[15] Above the cell's gate is the sign of Jupiter, whom, as the protector of such people, we will call upon for help with this oration:

A Petition to Jupiter[16] on Behalf of Solitary and Melancholic Madmen

This band of weaklings, deprived of all help and counsel, directed by your divinity, through me turns to you, O greatest son of Ops[17] and Saturn, brother and spouse of Queen Juno, justly called Jove because of the gifts[18] you bestow on the needy; called the Greatest Good because of the infinite goodness with which you govern the universe; called Satore,[19] Creator, High-Sounding, King of the Gods, Lord of the World, Rector of Olympus, Corrector of Vices and Crimes, Highest Ethereal Father, Sceptered One, Omnipotent One, and other illustrious epithets, because everything, at the slightest sign from you, is ready to obey. Therefore, being moved by such a great deity and awakened by such a majesty, I pray to you for that compassion which the Curetes showed toward you by nourishing you on Mount Ida,[20] so that you may have pity on these poor and disconsolate

---

[14] "Synagogue" both in the sense of a Jewish congregation and also in the broader sense of "collection." Garzoni used the term in this dual sense in his "Synagogue of the Ignorant", *La Sinagoga de gl'ignoranti* (Venezia: G.B. Somasco, 1589). Cherchi, 269, n. 11. The "Synagogue" is available in Garzoni, *Opere*. See also the Introduction, p. 7 and note 24.

[15] Garzoni evokes the famous description by Virgil *(Aeneid,* 6. 34ff) of Aeneas' consultation with the prophetess prior to his descent into Hell.

[16] Jupiter's epithets are in Giraldi, *De deis gentium,* 75–117.

[17] "Ops," goddess of riches, plenty, and fertility.

[18] "gifts," or *giovamento,* from Jove, or Jupiter, "jove-ness," or "helpfulness."

[19] Although Garzoni has "Satore" here, the more traditional epithet for Jupiter is "Stator."

[20] When Rhea gave birth to Zeus, she entrusted him to the Curetes and the nymphs Adrasteia and Ida. They fed him with milk from the goat, Amaltheia.

people. And if the love of Europa and of your sweet page, Ganymede,[21] fills your heart with joy, recalling the jealousy you felt, the suffering you went through, and the anguish which you endured, later surpassed by much greater pleasure that subsequently ensued, for the sake of that same enjoyment, I entreat you to bring joy to these afflicted ones, comfort these distressed ones, and deliver these melancholics out of their anguish and grief—these who are assigned to you as their favorable star.

If you are the one who gave birth to Minerva, Goddess of Wisdom,[22] purge their heads of all that insipidness which so abounds there. If you are truly the one called Panompheus because you hear everybody's voice, then hear and listen—not to their voices, but to the shrill cries of these abandoned ones. If you are the Hospital Jupiter, so celebrated by the poets, take care of these souls who, in this hospital, shout out loud for your help. If you are that Jupiter Penetrator, so beloved by the ancients, let these men's miseries penetrate not just the ears but even to the heart's core of such a compassionate god. If you are the Jupiter Stoneworker whose works are marvels in stone, what greater miracle could you perform than this: to remove from these insensible stones the savage and obdurate humor that possesses them?

If you are that Jupiter whom all men call "Genius," because of the genius and temperament you have of bestowing favors on all, I pray you, favor these—who have the greatest need of it—with a little bit of your blessing. If you are that Prodigious Jupiter who has performed so many miracles in former ages, now perform this one: that thorns may become roses, thistles become narcissuses, and nettles become fodder. Then, with merry voices, the whole Hospital will resound: "Long live great Jupiter Elicius, Anxurus, Aegiuchus, Lycaeus, Dodonaeus, Latialis, Dictaeus, Praedator, Ultor, Pistor, Ammon, Eleus, Cynethius, Atabyrius, Casius, Eleutherius, Nicephorius, Papeus, Lucetius, Olympius, Labradeus, Laprius, Maleaeus, Assabinus, Orceus, Larisseus, Enaesimus, Pulvereus, Triphylius!"[23] And singing solemn songs, they will all run to your temples, offering a thousand bunches of wild rue to your image because you will have purged them of all of the wildness that ruled over them.[24]

Therefore, confident as I am of your customary Jove-ness, I anticipate the appropriate aid and assistance for these sick ones.

---

[21] Garzoni reminds Jupiter of two rather sordid episodes of his love-life. Europa, the daughter of Phoenix, was raped by Jupiter in the form of a bull. Ganymede, a lovely boy, was also taken by Jupiter.

[22] Compare with the prayer to Minerva at the end of Discourse 2.

[23] Cherchi corrected several spellings of these epithets (271, nn. 19–26).

[24] According to custom, one of the sacred symbols of Jove was wild grass. The grass had medicinal properties and was used as an antispasmodic and hypotensive agent: Barelli, 41, n. 34.

The Fourth Discourse:
The Lazy and Good-for-Nothing

Among the race of madmen, it is good to include certain lazy and good-for-nothing men who always seem to be asleep when it comes to dealing with their affairs, displaying astonishing slothfulness, just as in the proverb of Diogenianus where he confirms that they sleep the sleep of Epimenides.[1] They demonstrate in their actions and affairs not, I would say, uncouthness, but rather negligence, inertia, and profound sleepiness. It may well be said of these men that which is affirmed about the Cimmerians who are overshadowed with such obscurity and darkness that bright Phoebus has banished himself from their minds forever.[2] So Homer said of these people:

Illos haud unquam radiis sol aspicit ardens,
Nec quando astriferum curru petit arduus axem,
Nec rursum ad terras magno devectus Olympo.

Nor does the bright Sun glance at them ever with his rays,
Neither when he climbs up the starry heaven
Nor yet when he returns again from heaven to earth.[3]

---

[1] In Manuzio, *Adagia* (392) and Erasmus, *Adagia*, 1.9.64: *dormis ultra Epimenidem*. Epimenides was a Greek sixth-century B.C. philosopher. As a boy, he fell asleep while looking for a sheep, and slept for fifty-seven years. Both Cherchi (271, n. 1) and Fiorato (n. 161) argue that Garzoni's text has erroneously attributed the story to a Diogenianus, while Erasmus clearly attributes the story to Diogenes Laertius.

[2] See Erasmus, *Adagia*, 2.6.34 (33: 307-8). "*Cimmeriae tenebrae*," or "Cimmerian gloom." Erasmus explains: "The adage takes its rise from the legendary darkness of the country of Cimmeria: [it is] shrouded in mist and cloud, nor does the bright Sun ever shine upon it but a dread night spreads over all." Also in Tixier, *Officina*, 7:48. Phoebus is the sun personified. Also in Manuzio, *Adagia* (644).

[3] Homer, *Odyssey*, 11:14-16. Garzoni's quotation of Homer in Latin may have come from Erasmus: see previous note.

Among these we have reason to place Vatia, a citizen of Rome, the only example used by Seneca in his *Epistles* of a good-for-nothing fool.[4] As he grew old with his slothfulness, he gave birth to a proverb: when people speak of a truly lazy, good-for-nothing fool, they would say, "*Vacia hic situs est,*" or, "Here lies Vatia."

Ovid also seems to allude to these men when he says:

Stulte quid est somnus gelidae nisi mortis imago?[5]

Fool, what is sleep but the image of icy death?

For, truly, a madman of this sort is so sleepy-headed in his actions that one can say that he is almost dead. So Dante, regarding these miserable folks, wrote the following verses *a propos* of them:

Fama di loro il mondo esser non lassa.
Misericordia et giustizia gli sdegna,
Non ragionar di lor, ma guarda, e passa.

The world will never let them have any fame;
Mercy and justice hold them in disdain.
Don't talk of them; only look and then pass by.[6]

But if modern examples have greater force in revealing these unhappy ones to the world, we can note the singular example of Cauccio of San Lupidio. He went to a tavern in Sinigallia, and while his companions ate a merry meal and sat at the table for two hours, he spent two and a quarter hours tying one of his shoestrings. When the host, thinking that he had dined with the rest, announced that it was time to go to bed, he asked for an awl so that he could make a new hole for his shoestring, because it seemed to him that his shoe still didn't fit him well enough.

But the case of Marchetto from Piombino is no less famous. On his way to Rome to seek a master in order to learn a trade so that he could make a living, he came upon a stone that he began to kick in front of him along the way. But before he had reached the nearest gate of Rome, he met all of his companions who had left with him and who were already returning, while he was still laboring to push the stone forward. So, in their presence, he finally put it in his pocket and said

---

[4] "Vacia": probably the consul, Servitius Vatia, who defeated the Sicilian pirates and the Isaurians. He is mentioned by Seneca in the *Epistles*, 55.4: Fiorato, n.165. Also in Tixier, *Officina* 6.67.

[5] Ovid, *Art of Love*, 2.9.41-42.

[6] Dante, *Inferno*, 3.49-51.

that when he arrived at the Roman wall, he would smash the stone against it in such a way that it would never again annoy travelers who were going to Rome.

Now these miserable and unfortunate subjects, devoid of wit and understanding, having need of Apollo's illumination, keep his sign above their cell as their guardian, while they remain holed up in the obscurity of this dreary hospice of their madness. Therefore, with solemn orations, we invoke the assistance of the divine Apollo to help them.

An Oration to the Divine Apollo on Behalf of Lazy and Good-for-Nothing Fools

O Sacred Apollo,[7] called Phoebus by the Greeks, who, with your golden mane, comfort and bring joy to both the hemispheres, welcomed by all, discourteous to none, cast the light of your divine beams on this blind and good-for-nothing gang of fools so that, because of you, they will feel that their minds have been illuminated. And by profiting from your god-granted illumination, may that virtue be exalted which killed the arrogant Cyclops, shot the iniquitous sons of Niobe, and wiped out that wretched serpent Python (because of which you were given the name Pythius, to your glory). Help, Lover of the River Amphrysus,[8] Resident of Mount Parnassus, Lover of Helicon,[9] Lord of the Caballinian Fountain,[10] Patron of the Laurel, Inventor of the Harp, Master of Astrology, and Prince of Physicians, help these poor Good-for-Nothing Madmen who have need of internal remedies to shed light on their sick brains, on their impoverished wit, on their obfuscated understanding, and on their lost memory.

And since you are called Pornopius[11] because you freed the Boeotians from mosquitoes, and Lemius because you cured the Sicilians from the plague, and Erethibius because you healed the Rhodians of their hemorrhoids,[12] therefore

---

[7] For these epithets, Garzoni follows Giraldi, *De deis gentium,* 7. 217ff.

[8] Amphrysus, where Apollo fed the flocks of King Admetus.

[9] Helicon: mountain in Boeotia, famous for its pure air, abundant water, fertile valleys, dense shade, and beautiful forests. There were statues to Apollo and the Muses on its summit.

[10] The fountain of Hippocrene, consecrated to the Muses. The fountain was struck out of Mount Helicon in Boeotia by the hoof of the winged horse Pegasus. Pegasus appears in several Greek myths, most notably in the story of how Bellerophon, on Pegasus' back, defeated the Chimaera and the Amazons single-handedly.

[11] Giraldi, *De deis gentium,* has both "Pornopius" and "Pronopius." In Strabo (*Geography*) Apollo is reported to have freed the Boeotians of locusts.

[12] Strabo, *Geography* (6:127) explains that the Rhodians, who call *erysibê erythibê,* have a temple of Apollo Erythibius in their country. Strabo indicates that Apollo cured the Rhodians of a type of mildew. Garzoni seems to be playing with the fact that the same word, *marovelle,* means both "mildew" and "hemorrhoids."

I pray that to these noble titles, which correspond to your great godliness, and those other titles—Thymbraeus, Cataon, Cyllaeus, Teneatus, Larissenus, Tilphosius, Leucadius, Phylleus, Libyssinus, Smintheus, Pataraeus from Patara in Lycia, Cynthius from Cinthus in Delos, Cyrrhaeus from Cyrrhea, Clarius from Claro in Colophon, Lycius from Lycia, Grynaeus from that forest in Ionia, Marmarinus from Marmarino Castle, that it may please you to add to these epithets one other—Physician to the Good-for-Nothings—so that your name may be extolled with great praises throughout the whole world. But if you, with compassion, care for these folks, just as you did for the populations mentioned above, you will see consecrated to your image in the temple at Delphi a pair of high-powered spectacles of sixty diopters[13] as a true sign of your having cared for and healed such senseless people as these. And this one honor will always be attributed to you: that blind men see light because of Apollo's spectacles on their noses. So hasten with your succor, because even the slightest delay in helping them will cause these lazy fools to become totally stupid.

---

[13] Indicating very high-power lenses. See Garzoni, *La piazza universale* (Venice: G.B.Somasco, 1586), Discourse 64, "Occhialari," or "Optician": Cherchi, 274, n. 11.

The Fifth Discourse:
The Drunkards

It is an obvious fact, well known to everyone, that among the various types of substances is the one caused by the fumes and vapors of wine, which gives rise to that type of madmen whom we commonly refer to as drunken fools. They have this characteristic: that when they are touched and warmed up by wine, they raise such a tumult and roar that they resemble Sterope and Bronte in Vulcan's furnace.[1] Because of this, the philosopher Athenaeus, in the fourteenth book of his *Deipnosophists*,[2] posed this question: why is it that the poets imagine that Dionysius or Liber are insane? He answered this question in the first chapter in this way: "My friend Timocrates, many people believe Dionysus to be insane because those who abuse wine become rowdy."[3] Ovid also touched on this issue:

Iurgia praecipue vino stimulata caveto,
Et nimium facile ad fera bella manus.

Above all, beware of conflicts caused by wine
And of hands too quick to do battle. [4]

On this topic, Herodotus said,

---

[1] Two of the three Cyclopes who lived in Vulcan's furnace, personifications of thunder and lightning.

[2] Athenaeus's *Deipnosophists* (ed. and trans. Charles Breton Gulick [London: Putnam's, 1927]) in thirty books, was edited by Aldo Manuzio in 1514 and reprinted several times in the sixteenth century. Natale Conti prepared a Latin translation of the work, first published in 1556 (*Athenaei Dipnosophistarum* . . . [Lyons: Faure, Jacques Honorat, Barthelemy, 1556]). The *Deipnosophists* is a summary of knowledge of science, especially of botany: 6.7. This magical agglomeration of all sorts of miscellany is one of Garzoni's chief sources. See *Athenaeus and his World*, ed. D. Braund and J. Wilkins (Exeter: University of Exeter Press, 2000).

[3] Athenaeus, *Deipnosophists*, 6: 303: "The majority of writers, friend Timocrates, call Dionysus 'the mad' from the fact that most people who take a pull at unmixed wine grow uproarious."

[4] Ovid, *Art of Love*, 1.591–592

Vino in corpus descendente, mala verba et insanientia educuntur.[5]

When wine goes down into the body, bad and foolish words come out.

Xenophon, too, giving good counsel to the great Captain Agesilaus[6] regarding abstinence from wine said,

Abstine ab ebrietate, atque ab insania,

Abstain from drunkenness as you would from madness,

making no distinction between a drunk man and a madman, because when the vapors of wine ascend to the brain, they steal sight, knowledge, and judgment and instantaneously crush all of the most noble faculties of the soul.

Saint Ambrose touched beautifully on this topic in his book, *On Fasting:*

Cum ebrii fuerint de continentia disputant, ubi unusquisque pugnas suas enarrat, ibi fortia facta praedicat, vino madidus et somno dissolutus, nescit mente, quid lingua proferat.[7]

When they are drunk, they argue about temperance, and when they all recount their battles, they boast of their valiant acts. So, dead drunk and incoherent from sleepiness, the mind does not understand what the tongue speaks.

On the same subject, in the *Decretals,* the thirty-ninth distinction, are written these valuable words:

Alienum est a sapiente comessationibus, potationibus et ebrietatibus vacare.[8]

It is foreign to the wise man to partake of feasting, libations, and drunkenness.

Our Poet, Dante, greatly praises that first Saturnian age when people would not go to taverns to take the cork from the barrels, but instead ran to the rivers to drink fresh water out of their hands, saying:

That first age was as fine as gold,
When acorns were made luscious by sharp hunger,
And every brook made honey-sweet by thirst.[9]

---

[5] Athenaeus, *Deipnosophists*, 6: 303. Not in Herodotus, *Histories.*

[6] Athenaeus, *Deipnosophists*, 6: 305. Agesilaus II (438–c. 361 B.C.) was king of Sparta and scholar.

[7] Ambrose, *De Elia et ieunio,* PL 14.715.

[8] Gratian, *Decretum*, Distinction 44, "*Cum autem vinolentus*": PL 187.227 CD.

[9] Dante, *Purgatorio*, 22. 148–150.

How blessed our age would be, were it adorned by such abstinence the way that age was! But the fact is, you can't find anything but sauced-up magpies, chattering like fifty, as soon as the elixir of Lyeus[10] begins to take effect.

A single example from our time will fill the whole world with laughter. If Margute dal Binasco[11] drinks just three glasses of muscatel, not having cured himself of Bacchus, with his brains racing at full speed, he arrives in Cuccagna with the first post and concurs with King Panigone[12] at the first opportunity, and he looks like the merriest companion on earth. But when the Vernaccia touches the peak of his noggin, he becomes like one of the Maenads,[13] running around the house, and raises so much havoc in every place, that it looks as if Baiardo[14] had broken from his harness, as no one would dare get in the way of such a headstrong beast. But sometimes he treats the company to great enjoyment and pleasure, such as the night when, being drunk and going to bed, he gazed at the moon and, thinking it was a river, said to his friends and companions, "Hold onto me, I pray you, so that I don't drown myself in this river!"

Among the ancients, the Scythians and the Thracians are criticized because their greater glory rested on their drinking so much that they became drunk. So Horace wrote of them,

Natis in usum laetitiae
scyphis pugnare Thracum est.[15]

Tussling with the goblets kept for pleasure
is characteristic of the Thracians.

And Aristotle, in reproaching the Syracusans,[16] writes that they would go on, day after day — sometimes for ninety days — in this predicament of daily drunkenness, considering it a noble and glorious practice.

It has been written of Tiberius Nero that, above all others, he was so dedicated to drunkenness that he was shamefully called, instead of Tiberius, "Biberius,"

---

[10] "Lyaeus," one of Bacchus' epithets, meaning "Loosener." Pliny, *Natural History* ,10.58–59 discusses drunken parrots and magpies.

[11] Binasco: small town a few miles south of Milan.

[12] King Panigone. Cherchi wonders if Garzoni is referring to Rabelais' character, Pantagruel, although there is apparently no Italian source for this reference: 276, n. 13. However Fiorato, n. 192, believes the reference is to "Panicone," described in Battaglia as "a corpulent loafer and pig." This profile corresponds well with the imaginary King of Cockaigne, frequently associated with Pantagruel, who, in the fourth book of Rabelais, Chapter X, receives Panurge royally in a courteous atmosphere.

[13] Maenads: followers of Bacchus.

[14] Baiardo or Bayard, Rinaldo's horse in Ariosto's *Orlando Furioso*.

[15] Horace, *Carmina*, 1.27. 1–2; Tixier, *Officina*, 5.51.

[16] *Politics*, 5.10.

"The Drinker": instead of "Claudius," he was called "Caldius," or "The Cauldron": and instead of "Nero," he was called "Mero," or "Pure Wine."

But whoever does not know what a great evil drunkenness is, has only to read the poets' descriptions of Bacchus, for this will clarify the reader's error once and for all. For Bacchus was depicted in the form of a baby boy because drunks lose their wits and understanding, and in the form of a woman because drunkards are incapable of any manly act, and undressed or naked, because you may not tell a drunk anything that you may want to be kept secret; and drawn in a chariot, because in the inebriated one finds a wondrous instability and volubility; and with a garland of vines around his head because just as vines bring down a wall, so are drunks capable of all sorts of destruction.

Enough has been said about this race of fools, who show the sign of the god Abstemius[17] above their cell in this Hospital, because he is the protector and advocate of all drunkards. So, for their assistance and favor, let us turn to him with the following oration:

An Oration to the God Abstemius on behalf of Drunken Madmen

With few words, but with so much more ardor, I do not come to you in a moment of such dire need, O you, disdainful of Lyeus, adversary of Bacchus, foe of Liber, and mortal enemy to Bromius,[18] praying to you, by the virtue which made you cause the Locresians[19] to maintain that getting drunk with wine was a capital offense, and prodded the sophists Moschus and Apollonius of Tyana[20] to think thoughts that are so distant and removed from wine, namely that they hated the Phigalians[21] more than they hated sickness, because they did not know how to live outside of a tavern. I pray that you assist these men in turning from their mad craving to be drunk all the time. If you grant them this grace and favor,

---

[17] Abstemius, a deity not located in the traditional pantheon; perhaps invented by Garzoni. Ironically, the name of this god of drunkards evokes "abstinence."

[18] Lieo, Liberus, Bromius: all epithets of Bacchus. Giraldi, *De deis gentium*, 152.

[19] Locresians: Greek settlers of Locres or Calabria.

[20] Moschus and Apollonius of Tyana: Greek rhetoricians. The first, Moschus of Elis, drank only water: Athenaeus, *Deipnosophists* 1:191. Apollonius of Tyana was born in Cappadocia in the fourth century B.C. He was thought to have magical and supernatural powers such as being able to raise the dead and heal the sick. In Philostratus' biography, he is depicted as having parallels to Christ. Garzoni's source is Tixier, *Officina*, 5.50, *On Sobriety and Abstinence*.

[21] Phigalians: residents of Phigalia, in Arcadia, known for their dread of epidemics which they would drown in wine: Athenaeus, *Deipnosophists,* 7:48, and Celio, *Lectiones*, 712: 1069.

we vow—here and now—that we will hang before your image a little flask of perfect ribolla from Zante[22] as a sign of the health you have brought to this mad rabble who need brains more than wine. Peace be with you, and help those who need your help.

---

[22] "ribolla from Zante": a wine from the Ionian island of Zante.

The Sixth Discourse:
The Forgetful and Demented

Among modern physicians, John Fernelius Ambianus,[1] in defining what dementia is, writes these exact words:

> *Amentia est, vel imaginationis, vel mentis occasus, atque privatio qua iam ab ipso ortu perculsi affectique vix inopia mentis loqui discunt.*

> Dementia is an obfuscation of the imagination or mind and such a serious impairment that those who are afflicted with it from birth can barely learn to speak because of the poverty of their minds.[2]

And he continues,

> *Huius classis est fluxa et amissa memoria.*

> A fluid or lost memory belongs to this category.[3]

This loss of memory produces those types of fools that we usually term forgetful or demented. They are easy to recognize by this: their discourse is incoherent and they lack even the least scintilla of a capacity to reflect, demonstrating the truth of that line in Galen in the preface to his book *On Sects:*

> *Memoriam commendat magna et frequens rerum meditatio.*

> Intense and frequent reflection calls on memory.

It is quite true that this sort of madness can be caused by a defect of nature or from an extraordinary accident during adulthood, as examples from various authors testify to all. Celio, among others, writing about those who have lost their

---

[1] See 56 n. 8 above.
[2] Garzoni uses dementia to refer to a variety of organic brain disorders including brain damage resulting from birth trauma.
[3] Ambianus, *Pathologia*, 5:2 (504). Jean Fernel (1497–1558), professor of medicine at Paris: Fiorato, n. 105. See also the Introduction, 16–17.

memory through accidents, says that Messalla Corvinus,[4] an outstanding orator in his time, lost his memory two years before he died so that he was not able to string together four words on the same topic nor make good sense to the soul and the mind of his listener.

Bibaculus[5] wrote that the same thing happened to Orbilius of Benevento,[6] the one whom Cicero calls "The Wounding Master of his Students."[7] Among those who, by nature, were barren of memory, Cicero sets forth the example of Curio the Elder[8] who was so lacking in memory that at certain times, in court, he forgot what the litigation was all about.

Seneca writes of Calvisius Sabinus[9] that he was, by nature, endowed with such a weak memory that he would sometimes forget the names of Ulysses or Priam or Achilles, even though they had previously been fixed in his mind.

The marvelous madness concerning the memory of Coroebus, son of the Phrygian, Mygdon, is celebrated by Lucian and Eustathius. He tried to count the infinite numbers of waves in the sea, even though, by nature, he couldn't count past five.[10]

---

[4] M. Valerius Messalla Corvinus, orator and Roman general (64 B.C.-8 A.D.) who fought in the civil wars. The example is in both Tixier, *Officina*, 4.7 and Celio, *Lectiones*, 410.

[5] M. Furius Bibaculus, b. 103 B.C. Roman satirist. Classed by Quintilian along with Catullus and Horace as one of the most distinguished Roman poets. Garzoni may be referring to his poem about the loss of memory of Orbilius Pupillus.

[6] Orbilius Pupillus from Beneventum, Latin grammarian who was Horace's teacher, who commented on his strictness in his letters (*Epistles*, 2. 1. 70). The anecdote is in Tixier, *Officina*, 4:7.

[7] The epithet is not from Cicero, but from Horace, *Epistles*, 2.1.

[8] Curio: C. Scribonius Curio. Seneca (*Ad Lucilium* 27 [1:195]) reports that he hired slaves to learn Homer and Hesiod by heart so that they could prompt him when he tried to entertain guests with quotations from those authors. He was a senator and Roman consul (first century B.C.), a good friend of Cicero (*Brutus* 110, 122, 216; *De Oratore* 2.98) who said of him that he had only one of the faculties of a great orator: elocution. He lacked memory and was ignorant without being aware of it. He was nevertheless appointed *pontifex maximus* in 53 B.C.

[9] Calvisius Sabinus, in Tixier, *Officina*, 4:7 and in Celio, *Lectiones*, 505. Sabinus was a wealthy contemporary of Seneca (see *Ep.* 27). He was considered ignorant but longed to be thought of as a learned man.

[10] Coroebus: young Trojan hero, and son of Mygdon, lover of Cassandra. He is mentioned by Virgil (*Aeneid*, 2.341, 386, 407, and 424). Also in Tixier, *Officina*, 5.32. The anecdote is also the basis for Erasmus's adage, "*Stultior Coroebo*," or "As foolish as Coroebus": *Adagia*, 2.9.64 (34:114). Lucian does not report the anecdote, only referring to Coroebus as a very gullible fool (*Erotes* 53). The story of Coroebus evokes another of Erasmus's adages, "*undas numeras*" or"You are counting the waves": 1.4.44 (31:354). Eustathius mentions Coroebus together with Melitidis and Mammacutus as examples of fools in his commentary on verse 552 of Homer's Odyssey: Eustathius, *Commentary* (Leipzig: Wiegel, 1825), 395.

For our last example, Pliny tells how the Thracians are so obtuse and their memory so flighty that they cannot count beyond four.[11] He also swears that Atticus, the son of Herodes the Sophist,[12] had such a shabby memory that he could not retain in his mind the rudiments or the first letters of the alphabet.

And the cause of all this—according to the physicians—is a tempest of the mind which makes all of the functional centers of the brain full of torpor and sloth—to describe it in their terms—and therefore they are unable to retain anything in their minds.

The case of Melchior of Rivabassa is a notable example of this in our time. In his days, he appeared to be so forgetful and demented that whenever anybody asked him his mother's or father's name he was incapable of remembering them. This is the same clumsy Melchior who one day, during a fair in Bergamo, asked his friend whether or not the Jews were Christians.[13]

There is yet another example, just as ridiculous, of Marchetto of Tolentino.[14] He had been invited to lunch by some gentlemen of Foligno, but because of his age, he lacked teeth for chewing. He forgot the artificial teeth that he occasionally used, securing them in place with silver wire. So he returned home to look for them, and turned everything topsy-turvy—even his huge corn crib, certain that he had left them there.

So these are the forgetful and demented fools who have been assigned a room in our Hospital that we call the Chamber of Oblivion. On their door hangs the image of Charon, a god favorable and propitious for their needs. It is Charon whose help I request for their aid and assistance, with the oration that follows:

---

[11] Aristotle, *Problems*, 15.3 reports that the Thracians "alone among men" count in fours "because their memory, like that of children, cannot extend further and they do not use a large number of anything."

[12] Atticus: Athenian rhetorician, son of the sophist Tiberius Claudius Atticus Herodes; b. 104 A.D.-d. c. 180.

[13] Melchior is an example of madness in one of Garzoni's contemporaries.

[14] Tolentino: town in the Marches.

An Oration to Charon[15] on Behalf of Forgetful and Demented Madmen

Now I turn to you, old Charon, Prince of the Stygian Lake, Lord of Cocytus, famous Helmsman of Lethe, Principal Keeper of Phlegethon![16] For the sake of that boat which transports mortals over the Waters of Oblivion, I pray you bring back this group of forgetful ones, who, having lost the memory of earthly things, are immersed, or rather immobilized, in the waters of Lethe right up to their chins. If you help this demented rabble, you will see, in front of your bearded image, in the temple consecrated to your name in the land of the Cyzicenians,[17] a cage full of crickets as a sign of having helped these fools who have less memory than a cricket, but will then demonstrate so much of it that "Blessed be Charon for that glory!"—as long as you remember to pull them from the Lethean slime where they have been buried for eternity. So turn the rudder of your boat and ferry them back now, while your memory of this supplication is fresh, for the need is greater than it has ever been.

---

[15] Charon, god of the Underworld, He transported the dead across the River Styx or the River Lethe where they lost all memory of their past lives. Charon's epithets and attributes are derived from Giraldi, *De deis gentium*, 7 (215–16). Folegno, *Baldus*, also contains several references to Charon.

[16] Phlegethon, river of the Underworld, in which flames, not water, flowed. See Brumble, *Myths*, 295–98, esp. 297.

[17] Cyzicenians, inhabitants of the island of Cyzicus off the coast of Mysia, named after Cyzicus, a son of Apollo. They are the subject of an adage, "*Cyziceni staters*," or "Cyzicene staters": Erasmus, *Adagia*, 3.1.73 (34:210). In Tixier, *Officina*, 2.109.

The Seventh Discourse
The Dumb, Vacant, and Lifeless

Those who—because of their actions, words, deliberations, and resolutions—seem like immovable and insensible stones deserve to be counted among the pantheon of madmen. We assign them the names dumb, vacant, and lifeless, since they are practically like the dead in all of their operations.[1]

Included in this race were the Gamphasantes,[2] inhabitants of a region of Libya, who had such a fearful and death-like temperament that they ran from meeting anyone, nor could they force themselves to be in a social situation, since they felt lost in the company of others.

The ancient Reggians are also described as being of this temperament. Because of their sloth and amazing shyness, they gave rise to a saying. When men spoke of a lost and, by all rights, dead man, they would say *Rheginis timidior*, that is, "More bashful than the Reggians."[3]

Who would deny that Artemon,[4] the Greek, was a dumb fool and truly vacant? For no reason, he remained holed up in his house between two walls and had two of his servants continually hold an iron shield over his head so that nothing would hurt him by falling on him from above. When he would occasionally go out of his house, he was carried on a stretcher with a regally-appointed roof over it in order to counter the same fear.

---

[1] Garzoni's epithets for this variety of madness, "dumb, vacant, and dead," do not clearly convey the nature of the disorder he is describing. The examples he gives here are all cases of what would be termed phobias today, most of them social phobias.

[2] Gamphasantes: people of Ganamantes, in Libya. Herodotus (*Histories*, 4.174) says that they were people who avoided others and all society at all cost, and compared them to the Troglodytes. Tixier, *Officina*, 4:48.

[3] Erasmus, *Adagia*, 12.9.27 (34:100). Also in Manuzio, *Adages* (716). Rhegium is the Latin name for Reggio in Emilia.

[4] Artemon. Identified by Fiorito as Arthemo(n), mentioned by Cicero, *Verrines*, 2.128. Also in Tixier, *Officina*, 7:48. In Pliny's *Natural History*, 28.2, he is described as a physician famous for his cruel and magical remedies.

What do Aristophanes and Lucian report about one Plutus?[5] He was so completely vacant that any little puff of wind made him tremble from head to foot.[6]

In our time, we have the memorable example of that man from Monferrato,[7] who was giving an oration to certain people. When he mounted the lectern, he shut his eyes, and, with his eyelids closed and his tongue warbling like a thrush, he could barely finish his introduction because he became so paralyzed.

And this happened to a certain Colombino from Bergamo, even though he was considered to have an excellent mind: while giving a speech, he repeated the same gesture many times, but his words stopped in mid-sentence. While the gestures were done with great fervor, the words were frozen and did not dare to come out, so that there was little correspondence between the one and the other.

Among our examples, I consider the case of that man from Salona[8] not unworthy of our attention. When he rose to the bar to plead his client's case, he was overcome by an icy cold sweat that put him into a tertian fever which sent him off — as if by the next post — to Rhadamanthys.[9]

Now these fools are properly recommended to the god Sentinus,[10] Protector of the Senseless, and in front of their cell in the Hospital, they have raised his insignia because they expect the aid from him which we earnestly seek through the following oration:

An Oration to the God Sentinus, on Behalf of the Dumb, Vacant, and Lifeless

O Patron of human sensibility, life and vigor of these limbs of ours and strength of our spirits! You who grant the dumb and vacant the courage that they need! From you these poor fools — dumb and vacant — anxiously await the appropriate

---

[5] Aristophanes, *Plutus*, 202–203. Plutus (the dispenser of riches) became fearful after Jupiter had blinded him so that he would not bestow gifts solely on the righteous. Also, Lucian, "Timon the Misanthrope," in *Lucian*, ed. Fowler, 1: 31–57.

[6] From Tixier, *Officina*, 5.29, "*De metu ac timore*." Also in Erasmus, *Adagia*, "*Timidus Plutus,*" 3.7.2.

[7] Monferrato: town in the Piedmont.

[8] Salona: possibly Salò, on the western shores of Lake Garda. Barelli (56, n. 8) argues that Solin, near Split on the Dalmatian coast, is meant.

[9] Rhadamanthys: a judge of the dead, known for his incorruptibility. He was the son of Zeus and Europa and brother of King Minos of Crete: Homer, *Iliad*, 14.332. He is also the subject of an adage: Erasmus, *Adagia*, 2.9.30 and 31 (34:101).

[10] Sentinus: Roman god who gave thought to infants at the time of their birth, and who therefore presided over human consciousness. See also Cherchi, 282, n. 8.

assistance! That courage which you gave to Theseus and Peirithous[11] so that they could penetrate the unrelenting shadows of the house of the god Dis; that same valor that you gave to Jason and Typhis[12] so they could plough the raging waves of the Colchian Sea—the first two to abduct the lovely Proserpine, the other two to steal the precious golden fleece; may that same courage be infused into them by your grace so that they may appear miraculously restored, to your glory and honor, from their fear, dumbness, and death. If they obtain this gift—as their hope promises them—they would want to dedicate to your glorious name a lovely bunch of nettles as an acknowledgement that their senses have been recovered with your prickly spurs and that their lost wits have been happily restored. Therefore, answer their prayers if this glorification touches you as it should.

---

[11] Theseus, the celebrated ancient hero and his friend. He is the subject of the adage, "Not without Theseus": Erasmus, *Adagia*, 1.5.27. Peirithous descended into Hades ("the house of the god Dis") to rescue Proserpine, whom Pluto had taken as his wife. Peirithous was killed, and Theseus was held there until rescued by Hercules: Tixier, *Officina*, 5.14 (719–20).

[12] Jason and Typhis: heroes who rescued the Golden Fleece.

The Eighth Discourse: The Round-Headed, Gross, and Simple-Minded

Those ignorant and uncivilized men whom everybody commonly calls Oxheads—who, because of their nature, can learn nothing, and are so brilliant that it is enough that someone tells them that a jackass is a parrot for them to believe it; they are the ones whom we presently call round-headed, gross, and simple-minded.

In this regard, Battista Egnazio[1] mentions a certain Britannione who was by nature so round-headed and silly that his teacher was never able to get into his head the smallest part of the alphabet.

Philonides of Malta, fat in body, sillier than a castrated calf, was so slow in learning anything that when one would speak about an out-and-out ox-head, they would use the proverb *"Indoctior Philonide,"* that is, "More ignorant than Philonides."[2]

In our time, we could look at Cecchone of Minerbio[3] to see notable stupidity. One day, he got the idea that Bolognese frosting[4] was made with butter, so he didn't want to eat it during a day of abstinence, while the others attacked the container, saying that they had previously been given a dispensation for such a prohibition.

Santuccio of Fermo showed himself to be even more fat-headed: when he was having a meal with some merry fellows at the port of Fermo,[5] he ate a sea-turtle

---

[1] "Battista Egnazio" (ca. 1473–1553), pseudonym of G.B. Cipelli, Venetian humanist and professor of rhetoric; adversary of Sabellico. He published with Aldo Manuzio commentaries on the classics as well as works of literature and history.

[2] Cherchi (283, n. 3) notes that both of these anecdotes are in Tixier, *Officina*, 4.11, where, however, the first story relates to the emperor Licinius, not to "a certain Britannione." Garzoni also refers to a "Britannione" in his *Synagogue*, where he is also describing an imbecile. The story of Philonides is also in Erasmus, *Adagia*, 2.6.30 (33:305) as well as Manuzio, *Adagia* (639). Erasmus reports that "he was pilloried in several places by Aristophanes as lecherous and lavish with toadies."

[3] Minerbio: small town between Bologna and Ferrara.

[4] Bolognese frosting: a sugary crust used to decorate sweets.

[5] Port of Fermo: Port of San Giorgio in Fermo on the Adriatic Sea.

thinking it was an oyster, and insisting to all of them that it was the very best oyster that had ever been seen at that port.

Castruccio of Rovigo proved to be no less silly, since he was easily persuaded that John the Priest (Prester John) was none other than the Parson of Bebbe.[6] And what is told of Scarlino of Viadana[7] is no less enjoyable. Once he believed that the bell-tower of the Cathedral at Pisa[8] had sailed all the way to Livorno and then sailed back to its proper place.

But the last one—regarding Andreuccio of Scarparia[9]—adds the last condiment to all the others. One time, he believed a friend who told him that five hundred Turkish galleys had been spotted in the forest of Baccano[10] and that they were heading for Rome to sack that city. But the pope's men, with forty thousand balloon pumps, had caused such a tempest that the ships were all dispersed and smashed to smithereens throughout the woods, and fragments could be found everywhere.

Of these *cermisoni*,[11] many are born in Valtolina and especially in Valcamonica.[12] They are so gullible that they believe whatever is told them. Like the one who thought that the Arsenal at Venice was a goblet boutique; another believed that the bell tower of San Marco had been banished to Lizzafusina[13] for ten years on suspicion that it had committed treason; another one, more fat-headed than an elephant, believed that the *Bucentoro*[14] had put on riding boots and galloped from Venice to Tripoli in Syria in one night.[15] Yet another whale believed that the Po River had taken the Brenta River for his wife, and as a result the

---

[6] Prester John or John the Priest, *il Prete Iani*, was a legendary figure of Eastern Christianity during the Middle Ages. He was the emperor of an ill-defined kingdom. The "Parson of Bebbe" is obscure, but no doubt a very minor figure, indeed, compared with the famous Prester John. Garzoni mentions the Parson of Bebbe again in his *Sinagoga*, 13.14. Cherchi, 284, n. 6.

[7] Viadana: small town on the Po, about 20 miles southwest of Mantua.

[8] The famous "Leaning Tower" of Pisa.

[9] Scarparia: possibly Scarperia, 15 miles north of Florence.

[10] Baccano: woods north of Latium, infamous for being a hiding-place for highwaymen. Mentioned in various places in Folegno, *Baldus*. Fiorato, n. 242.

[11] Cermisoni: perhaps a play on the name of Antonio Cermisone, famous physician and professor at the universities of Pavia and Padua: Cherchi, 284 n. 10.

[12] Valtolina (Valtelina) and Valcamonica: two Alpine valleys north of Bergamo and Brescia, respectively. Garzoni suggests that these valleys were so remote that their inhabitants could be easily duped.

[13] Lizzafusina: probably Frusina, small port south-west of Venice: Fiorato, n. 247.

[14] Bucentoro: see 57 n. 15 above.

[15] Tripoli in Syria: modern-day Tripoli, second city of Lebanon. It was a major port for travel between Europe and the Holy Land and Persia. The trip by sea would have taken many days.

Adige, his rival in love, was angry at the Po and vowed never to join waters with it again.[16]

Last of all, there is that prototypical jackass or camel who believed that Mount Baldo, near Verona,[17] went hunting one day and ran into some banished citizens. When he was stopped by them, he took up his giant crossbow and iron-tipped arrows and killed ten or twelve of them with one shot.

So these men have a cell in the Hospital over which hangs the insignia of the Egyptian Ox,[18] because it is to him, their protector and advocate, that they are commended. Therefore, with the following oration, I entreat him to assist and aid them.

An Oration to the Egyptian Ox on Behalf of the Round-headed, Gross, and Simple-Minded

These silly ox-heads, with great solemnity, turn to you, O Most Solemn Ox of the Egyptians, called Apis and Serapis by all, in order to obtain this favor from your hand: that, seeing that they are oxen just like you, you will be so beneficial to them that they may not one day grow so stupid that they are more stupid than camels.

Therefore, for that honor that is bestowed upon you in Egypt—which far exceeds that of the Tortoise worshipped by the Troglodytes, of the Viper, by the Fennians,[19] the Dove, by the Assyrians, the Stork, by the Thessalians, the Lioness, worshipped by the people of Ambracia, the Dragon, worshipped by the Albanians, the Weasel, worshipped by the Thebans, the Cow, worshipped by the Tenedians—I pray and again beseech you to grant unto them this requested grace and favor.[20]

If you do this for them—as we hope you will—you will see placed in the temple consecrated to you, before your image, a shock of May-harvested hay with a wooden hoe next to it, showing that these men, through your favor, continue in their oxen-like state and do not grow ever more stupid.

---

[16] Po, Brenta, and Adige: three rivers in the vicinity of Venice.

[17] Mount Baldo: a high mountain—approximately 6600 feet high—north of Verona. In his *Piazza*, Garzoni makes reference to the "Travels of Monte Baldo" (*Viaggio di Monte Baldo*) by Francesco Calzolari (Venice: Valgrisio, 1566).

[18] Egyptian Ox: the bull Apis. The Bull of Memphis, sun god of Egyptian mythology. According to Apollodorus (*Library*, 2.1.1) Serapis is the name of Apis after his death. Aelian, *On the Characteristics of Animals*, 12.40, reported that the 29 marks on the body of Apis represented a complete astronomical and physical system.

[19] Baltic people described by Tacitus, *Germania*, 48.

[20] This list of animal deities is found in Tixier, *Officina*, 1.10, "*De multitudine deorum*": Cherchi, 285, n. 13.

The Ninth Discourse:
The Idiots and Airheads

These unlucky, miserable wretches who, with the wind blowing through their heads, and their brains having shrunken to the point that their heads seem more like eggshells, and because of the flaws in their actions, words, and thoughts make everyone who sees or hears them burst out laughing, are, among the ranks of fools, termed idiots or vacuous ones.

In ancient times, the Bithynians[1] were found to be of this type because—as Celio writes—they would climb to the very tops of mountains and salute the moon and confabulate with it even though they never received any sort of reply from it.

The Boeotians[2] —according to the testimony of authors—also possessed this sort of madness, causing the poet Horace to write:

Boeotum in crasso iurares aere natum.

You would swear he was born breathing the thick air of Boeotia.[3]

Among modern examples, the case of Francino of Matelica[4] may prove sufficient. Not holding himself back from being even a little more vacuous, every morning he would take his mother's bobbin—she, an old woman of seventy years—and, seating himself in the sun, set himself to spinning flax into thread. But he would so ruin the flax and the linen that the old woman would become infuriated and was impelled to crack her bobbin over his head every time. So, ranting and raving, she despaired of her son, whom she thought had very little wit and understanding.

---

[1] Bithynians: inhabitants of Bithynia in Asia Minor. The example is in Celio, *Lectiones*, 708.

[2] The legendary stupidity of the Boeotians is found in Tixier, *Officina*, 7.48, Celio, *Lectiones*, 708, and Erasmus, *Adagia*, 2.3.7 (33: 134), "Boeotian brains," where Erasmus says, "The Boeotians had a bad reputation in Antiquity for their stupidity ... as a result, everything pointless and doltish was called Boeotian."

[3] Horace, *Letters*, 2.1.244.

[4] Matelica: town in the Marches.

Mateuccio of Valvasson, poor soul, was another of this type, because when his father sent him into the country to see what the harvesters were doing, even though he was grown up and thirty-four years old, he would get into playing Draw the Stick with the children, and spent the whole day occupied in such silliness.[5] He returned home without giving any account of his purpose to the one who had sent him there.

Another of this type was that one from the castle at Bubano in Romagna whose brain showed sympathy with the name of his town.[6] Once, being completely vacant, he was supposed to deliver food to some workmen on orders from his master, but instead he went into a wheat field and occupied himself making pipes and whistles like the ones children play. He spent the entire day in this foolishness while the workmen were expecting this dumbbell to arrive with their lunch and were starving to death.

But the example of Tonio Buffalora[7] is the icing on the cake. While he was returning from Rome and passing through the pine woods near Ravenna, he collected a satchel-full of flies and mosquitoes—the big ones that those pine woods produce in abundance. He also collected a large pocket-full of horse-flies. He took them all to his hometown, and as soon as he arrived, he notified all of his friends and relations that they should come and see him, for he wanted to make them a gift of the foreign and beautiful things he had brought back from Rome. They all knew he was a fool but hadn't thought he was really as bad as they soon discovered, because he took them all off to a private chamber where he released all of the flies, mosquitoes, and horse-flies which flew into their eyes and noses, causing such a disturbance that they all laughed and were truly ready to die laughing at the novelty of the thing.

So fools of this brood are called idiots or vacuous ones, and within our Hospital have for their sign the Samian Ewe[8] as their great benefactor. Therefore, in this, our oration, we will request her aid and succor.

---

[5] "Draw the Stick," a children's game similar to drawing straws, where the winner is the one who gets the longest stick: Cherchi, 287, n. 4.

[6] Perhaps a reference to a play on "Bubano" and "Bubalo" or "Bufalo," all sounding like *bue*, or ox, meaning "fool." Fiorato, 184, nn. 262 and 265.

[7] Another play on "buffalo," as above.

[8] Garzoni alludes to an anecdote in *Sinagoga*, 9.12. Mandrabulo, a Samian, would offer a sheep to Juno every year; the first year, he offered a sheep of gold, the second year, one of silver, and each year thereafter a cheaper one, just as this sort of fool's brain shrinks more and more every year: Cherchi, 287, n. 8. Samians were residents of the island of Samos in the Aegean Sea.

An Oration to the Samian Ewe on Behalf of the Idiots and Airheads

If the honor which the ancient Samians paid to you, O Venerable Ewe, is so great in itself that it far exceeds those which the Delphians paid to your enemy, the Wolf, and greatly surpasses those carried out in honor of the Roman Goose or the Egyptian Goat, and if the glorious worship of you is one of the most solemn rites that any people have ever celebrated, I now pray that, because of this honor and of that cult, you will take whatever care of these, your sheep, that you, being a sheep like them, consider appropriate. And furthermore, if you do not favor them in this hour of their need, you will lose their devotion for you and, easily revolting from the Ewe, they will turn their prayers toward the god Castrone.[9]

So if you assist them we will present an offering of sheep's milk cheese from Gualdo or Rimini[10] to your image, so that people the world over will speak in praise of you, and all exclaim: "Long live Sheep and the Sheep-headed!"

---

[9] Castrone: a castrated sheep, also a stupid person. The castrated sheep also appears in Alciati's *Emblemata Liber* (n. 2) where it is used as an emblem of the Bituriges, one of the founding families of Milan.

[10] Gualdo: town about 10 miles east of Ferrara, although there is also a Gualdo near Forli. Rimini: town on the Adriatic coast.

The Tenth Discourse: The Jerks and Giddies

There is a nest of a certain type of fool that common folk usually call dazed or dizzy. They are known by these characteristics: they never do things according to the clock; they never speak to the issue; they never do anything with decorum; they never speak in a way that befits the situation, and they are so inept with every phrase, expression, word, gesture, or act that it is right that everyone should call them Jerks and/or Giddies.

In this regard, Cicero, in the second chapter of his *On Oratory*, describes the nature and properties of someone like this:

> *Qui tempus quid postulet, non videt, aut plura loquitur, aut se ostentat, aut eorum, cum quibus est, vel dignitatis, vel commodi rationem non habet, aut denique in aliquo genere, aut inconcinnus, aut multus est, is ineptus dicitur.*[1]

> He who does not see what the circumstances require either talks too much or makes an ostentatious display of himself, and has no idea of dignity or of what is appropriate for those around him; in sum, he is, in a certain sense, without elegance or is prolix or verbose; this is termed inept.

I would think that one could count the ancient, Amphistides—mentioned by Celio—among these fools. His brain was so dazed and dizzy that he didn't know whether or not he had been born to a father and mother, as is usually the case.[2]

Acesias, the physician, may also be counted among the dazed fools. This was his characteristic: that when he was treating someone, he always did the treatment in precisely the opposite way to that usually prescribed. Consequently, Paulus Manutius[3] devised this proverb:

---

[1] Cicero, *De Oratore*, 2.17.9.
[2] Celio, *Lectiones*, 843. Also in Tixier, *Officina*, 5:32 (775).
[3] Manutius, *Adagia*, 928.

Acesias medicatus est.

Treated by Acesias.[4]

Among those of our time, Franceschino of Montecuculo[5] was considered a great nut-case of this type who, acting in conformance with the name of his hometown, went into court to defend his client, and presented testimony and arguments that were totally adverse to the poor man.

A certain Ortensio of Sarni was also rebuked as a fool of this type by a judge in a certain lawsuit. He argued his case in perfect Ciceronian style, as far as the words went, but in every other respect, it was so bewildering and completely contrary to his purpose that the judge felt compelled to tell him that next time he had better bring to court the doggerel poems of Olimpio da Sassoferrato[6] and present them to him, because he would rather read them than his arguments *à la* Piovano Arlotto.[7]

Among the numbers of dazed and dizzy fools, a very great one is demonstrably that grocer from Castellina[8] who, instead of selling a servant-girl some starch, sold her some crystalline arsenic which almost caused her mistress to die from his error.

A certain servant called Lirone also showed himself to be an out-and-out stunned fool who, when he was told to skim a boiling cauldron, and not knowing what to do, threw out all of the broth, leaving the meat behind to dry out until the cook was ready to serve it.[9]

Bastiano of Monselice[10] was no less dazed. He was in the service of a certain Neapolitan Signor who ordered him to set out on the table some citrons and

---

[4] The adage is also in Erasmus, *Adagia*, 2.6.59 (33:321). According to Erasmus, the adage was applied to any condition which became progressively worse, and the more it was treated, the worse it got.

[5] Montecuculo: evokes "Mount Cuckoo," or "Stupidity Mountain." Located in the mountains north of Florence.

[6] Olympio da Sassoferato, or Olimpio degli Alessandri Baldassare: Dominican at the beginning of the sixteenth century and author of a half-dozen collections of poetry in the manner of Serafino Aquilano. His *Books of Love* contained strambotti, madrigals, dialogues, love letters, etc., published in the years 1530-1540, each with a woman's name as its title: Ficrato, 192, n. 277.

[7] Piovano Arlotto, the pseudonym of A. Mainardi (1396–1484), Florentine curate celebrated for his farces and popular comedies, *Facezie, fabule e motti del Piovano Arlotto*, ed. B. Pacini (Florence: B. Zucchetta, 1515). Fiorato, n. 278. A *piovano* is a local parish priest. See also Introduction, p. 9.

[8] Castellina: most likely the small town about 10 miles west of Parma.

[9] Garzoni mentions this Lirone in his *Piazza*, 93, dedicated to cooks. Cherchi, 290, n. 9.

[10] Monselice: about 10 miles south of Padua.

oranges. He went into the orchard and pulled out the best trees that they had, and brought them to his master in a bundle, along with considerable damage and no small amount of shame.

A similar example is that of another dazed fool from Bergamo who, commanded by his master to go up to the loft to get some wood for the fireplace, took a hatchet with him and began whacking at some beams that were holding up the roof. Eventually the master, noting the delay, forced him—by inflicting some good blows on him—to come back downstairs.

This other example, of Lucchino of Fusolara, is not unpleasing. He was in the service of a man who sold Malvasan wine. His master told him to pay careful attention to a gentleman who was a good friend of his. He told him that he should *sample* each of the barrels, but he thought that his master had told him to *smash* each of the barrels, so he picked up a lumberjack's axe and demolished more than four barrels before his master discovered his own error and his servant's stupidity.[11]

This one last example takes the prize. Bartolo of Calepio[12] near Bergamo, who was in the service of a very rich candle-maker in Venice, was watching his master make candles one day, and while the kettle was boiling and the wax was melting, he asked his master what was boiling in the kettle. Without cracking a smile, his master replied that it was sugar and honey to make marzipan. So this sweet-toothed idiot waited until his master had left, and picked up one of the pots in the shop and, before the wax had cooled and while it was still warm, he drank a pot-full, binding his teeth, tongue, and bowels together so that he almost died. Then, as he recounted the episode to his master, he, too, almost died from laughter, seeing how the dizzard had been taken in like that.

These, then, are the jerks and giddies who, in our Hospital, have the cell which displays outside it the sign of the goddess Bubona, the true friend of this type.[13] So, in the following oration, they are commended to her.

An Oration to the Goddess Bubona on Behalf of Jerks and Giddies

These Romagnan Geese, these castrated Apulian Lambs, these Marcanian Donkeys infinitely recommend themselves to you—Friend of Pan, Lady of the Flock, Shepherdess of the Herd, and Faithful Guardian of the Sheep-folds. They entreat you in the name of the love of Pasiphaë's Bull, of Aristo the Ephesian's Ass, of

---

[11] Luccino thought his master told him to smash (*spiana*) the wine casks, not simply taste them (*spina*).

[12] Calepio: town west of Milan.

[13] Bubona: Roman goddess of stables. Her special domain was the care of oxen and cows.

the shepherd Cratides' Goat,[14] and of the Mare so dearly beloved by Fulvius,[15] so that you will protect their flock as well, hardly different from the aforementioned beasts. And if it happens—as they hope it will—that you assume their protection, they intend to dedicate a farm-roasted buffalo to you and sing to you a beautiful hymn that includes your name, Bubona, and "buffalo" in every verse. Give your protection, therefore, to these buffaloes if you want the victim[16] to be consecrated to your honor and glory.

---

[14] Cratides, in Tixier, *Officina*, 5:46 (857).

[15] Garzoni evokes various animals associated with myths of zoophilia. For example, Pasiphaë made love to a bull. Tixier, *Officina*, 5:32 and in Plutarch, "Greek and Roman Parallel Stories," 29 in *Moralia*, 15 vols., trans. Frank Cole Babbitt (Cambridge, MA: Harvard University Press, 1962), 4:299.

[16] Victim: the sacrificed buffalo.

The Eleventh Discourse:
The Clumsy and Fatuous

There are certain unhappy wretches in the world, so dopey in their reasoning, so rude in their speech, so inept in their actions, activities, or transactions, that they rightfully earn the names of clumsy and fatuous fools in the eyes of the world, to distinguish them from all the other fools that we have listed above.

If we want to rely on the examples given by the ancient writers, we must say that Melitides, celebrated by Homer,[1] was one of these arch-clumsys because he arrived at Troy to give assistance after that city had already been destroyed and demolished. So he became proverbial in Lucian's phrase, "*Melitidis auxilium,*" or, "The assistance of Melitides," when one wishes to speak of succor given too late by a foolish and clumsy man.[2]

A certain Mamachutes was celebrated by Aristophanes because of these traits. Because he was so often cited by everyone because of his clumsy and dopey activities, from him comes the almost-proverbial phrase that we use: we term "Mamachutes" all those who are as clumsy and fatuous as he.[3]

This foolish disorder has been illustrated in the comedies of our time by Graziano of Bologna,[4] because when you hear a character like this conversing, you cannot imagine anything clumsier in the world. And his clumsiness has such power that it forces you to laugh out loud, because, in addition to the fact that

---

[1] Melitides is not mentioned by Homer. Garzoni's source is not known, but Melitides is mentioned by Eustathius, *Commentarii ad Homeri Odyssea*, 2 vols. (Leipzig: Weigel, 1825) in the context of a discussion of Odysseus' disregard for the dangers of the sea (1:395.52) where Mamacutus (see next paragraph) is also mentioned. Eustathius reports that Melitides could not count beyond four, and could not distinguish between his mother and father.

[2] Also in Tixier, *Officina*, 5:32, and Erasmus, *Adagia*, 4.4.69. In Lucian (*Erotes* 53), we find Melitides and Coroebus mentioned as examples of prototypical fools, but without further elaboration.

[3] Aristophanes, *Frogs*, 2. 989–991, where we also find reference to Melitides. Also Tixier, *Officina*, 5:32 (758); Celio, *Lectiones*, 630. From the Greek, literally, "hidden among his mama's skirts," i.e., stupid.

[4] Dr. Graziano, the mask of the fatuous physician-scientist of the Commedia dell'Arte. See 43 n. 16 above.

his speech is dull and his discourse is beyond all reason, and his conclusions are so out of sorts with their beginnings, and his gestures so disproportionate, and his voice coarse, and his actions so utterly crude, he arrives at certain conclusions that are so inept that they alone would cause anyone who was listening to them to choke with laughter.[5]

Giacomo of Pozzuolo is another one who makes our modern age illustrious with his clumsiness. When he walks, he looks like another crippled Aristogeiton;[6] when he speaks, one would think he had a frog in his throat; when he gesticulates, one would think that he was trying to mock both nature and art; when he recites anything, one would judge by his laughter that he was making light of the most serious matters; and when he discourses on any issue, you could not hear a funnier buffoon or a more ridiculous ass than he.

Then there is that oaf Andreuccio of Marano,[7] who, while reading from a legal notice that stated that certain fields had been rented for two hundred Venetian lira, said:

Moneta autem venetiana valebat ducentis libribus pro affitandis illis campibus.[8]

What can we say about that stupid pedant from Santo Arcangelo[9] who, translating into the vernacular this Latin phrase by Cato,

Cum ego Cato animadverterem quam plurimos homines errare in via morum,[10]

Because I, Cato, have realized that many err in their behavior,

made it:

Because I, Cato, knew full well that many men go wandering down the road of the Moors.

This conforms to what that other pedagogue said, expounding on that verse from Virgil:

---

[5] For example, "A Ferrarese is not a Paduan."

[6] Tixier (*Officina*, 3, *De homine: De claudicantibus*) explains that Aristogeiton feigned lameness to avoid military service.

[7] Marano: town 35 miles south-west of Bologna.

[8] Mangled Latin, "latino maccheronico," or macaronic Latin according to Cherchi, 292, n. 6. Andreuccio constructs his Latin from a mixture of Italian roots, vaguely plausible Latin endings, and approximations to Latin prepositions.

[9] Santo Arcangelo, probably Santarcangelo di Romagna, near Rimini.

[10] The phrase is the opening of the *Disticha de moribus* of Cato (Paris: S. Stephanus, 1557), 5.

Ille ego qui quondam gracili modulatus avena,[11]

I, the same person who once sang on a weak bagpipe,

translated it as

I, Giovanni Nicolò, who was condemned for the stinking crevices that I carried to Ravenna.

And what about that two-bit logician who translated this phrase by Pietro Hispano,

Barbara, Celarent, Darii, Ferro Baralipton

as follows:

The barbarous people of King Darius had put on their helmets, grumbling wildly.[12]

Then he translated this verse,

Celantes, Dabitis, Fapesmo, Frisesomorum

as

Those helmets gave both the Phrygians and the Moors spasms.

Coming to this verse,

Cesare, Camestres, Festino, Baroco, Darapti,

he rendered it as

Caesar's men had arrived at Mestre and were hurrying to beat him.

Finally, he came to this verse:

Felapton, Disamis, Datisi, Brocardo, Ferison,

---

[11] Virgil, *Aeneid*, 1, 1A, considered a spurious addition.
[12] This example and the next ones are taken from mnemonic devices for types of syllogisms created by Pietro Hispano (1220–1277), influential scholastic, physician, and Portuguese prelate who became Pope John XXI in 1276: *Summulae logicales*, 4.17: Cherchi, 293, n. 9. Our fool takes these lists of mnemonic names and tries to fashion a coherent sentence out of them. See T. Gilby, *Barbara Celarent* (London: Longmans, 1949).

which came out,

> Caesar said to Philip Anthony and to his friends to beat them with iron bars.

Wasn't Marinello of Villafranca[13] an obvious fool who wrote this address on a letter to one of his sons who was studying at the University of Bologna?

To the divine spirit of my son, Andrea Scarpaccia, who attends the school of the greatest physician in Bologna and who in three years will become another Falopia[14] if God, in his grace, attends to him in this life. In Bologna, near the Asinelli tower in the home of a woman who rents rooms.

So these are our clumsy and fatuous fools commended to the god Fatuellus,[15] advocate and — with sword drawn — defender of these sorts. Therefore, having the image of this god on the door of their cell, it is altogether fitting that we revere him with the following oration:

An Oration to the God Fatuellus, on Behalf of the Clumsy and Fatuous

May it please you, Great Monarch of the clumsy, phantasm of phantasms, because of the resonance of your name which conforms to your own genius, favor this clumsy band of fools who have turned pitifully to you. And in the name of that temple which you have in Valcamonica[16] where many fatuous ones merely depend on your dominion and command, these fools implore you that, even if your name means fatuous, at least you won't in fact be that way toward them.[17] And if you do that for them, they will offer up to your image one owl which will be a true sign that, through your intercession, they are no longer clumsy. This is your reward if you will be forthcoming and speedy with your assistance.

---

[13] Villafranca: perhaps Villafranca di Forli, just 8 miles from Bagnacavallo.

[14] Gabriele Falopia, or Falloppia, celebrated anatomist and surgeon (1523–1562). He was professor of anatomy at Padua: Fiorato, 204, n. 300.

[15] Fatuellus: god listed in Giraldi, *De deis gentium*, 426. Giraldi gives this as an epithet of Pan. Here Garzoni implies that his name is derived from "fatuous."

[16] See p. 48, note 23 and p. 86, note 12. This is Garzoni's third reference to these people.

[17] "fatuous" and "in fact": a play on these words, *fatuo and fatti*.

The Twelfth Discourse:
The Perverts

There are certain fools in the world who, together with the shrinkage of their brains and their loss of their senses, still retain certain vices which sometimes seem like they arise from a type of cunning which is in them, but in fact really follows more directly from defects in their corrupt and depraved minds rather than anything else. They resemble mules that kick anybody who comes near them because of their malicious nature. We were content with calling these sorts of men perverted madmen because we could not find a more appropriate and suitable word to apply to them.

Perhaps it would seem to some people that Cipius—written about by Lucilius[1]—could be placed among the group of perverted fools for this reason: because he allowed others to make use of his wife dishonestly; and he was a pervert because, not wanting it to appear to be voluntarily a cornucopia,[2] he feigned sleep while the adulterer—who was fully awake—wrestled with her in Venus's gymnasium.

That one in the hospital in Milan seemed no less of a perverted fool who summoned strangers to him, telling them that he wanted to show them the Valley of Jehosaphat.[3] Then, little by little he revealed to them his bare ass, causing all who came to see him to blush with embarrassment.

There was another one, even more perverted, who asked everyone if he could kiss them, and when they came close, he either smashed a chamber pot on their heads, sank his teeth into them, or did some other malicious thing.

The story is told of another perverted fool who, one day, standing at a window, saw a fair young maiden standing before him. As if he had instantly become

---

[1] Gaius Lucilius: Latin satirical poet, b. 148 B.C., d. 103 B.C., considered by some to be the writer who first gave form to the early satire. Horace (*Serm.* 1.10.64–72) criticized his hasty and careless writing, but admired his bold, fierce attacks and trenchant sharpness. Cicero, *Letters to His Friends*, 7.24.

[2] Cornucopia: meaning both a windfall or gift and also evoking a cuckold, from *cornuto*. Cipius was the subject of the adage "*Non omnibus dormio*," or "Not completely asleep": Erasmus, *Adagia*, 1.6.4. Also in Tixier, *Officina*, 7.

[3] Valley of Jehosaphat: traditional site of Mary's Assumption. A destination of pilgrims. According to Joel 3:2, it was also the site of the Last Judgement.

inflamed with love for her, he said to her, "Lady, do you feel love for me?" She replied, "No, Signor, because you are a Sir Mattio."[4] Then he replied, "Then let's get on with it!"

Regarding another perverted fool, this story has been told: One day, in the marketplace, he got up on a butcher's rack and gathered a ring of onlookers around him. He began to cry out so that everyone would come to hear him. Then, when the people had assembled, he said, "Imagine that I am the Great Beast who holds council with the other beasts. For my part, I want to go get some breakfast. The rest of you can go and become chopped meat."[5] And with that, he tricked everyone and left, to everybody's laughter and scorn.

This man was very much like another who entered the council chamber when certain serious matters regarding the city were being discussed and cried out in a loud voice, "I cast my *ballotta*; you're all *ballottas*."[6]

Norandino of Savignano,[7] a most perverted fool, was not unlike these. At a time when a great debate was being held in the town of Cesena, which is near his hometown, he happened to be going through the place where the disputants had gathered, and making room for himself with his heavy stick, he said, at the top of his voice, "I dispute this conclusion: that Savignano is not more than ten miles from Cesena, and furthermore, I hold that this is true: that Savignano is masculine and Cesena is feminine. And furthermore, I hold this to be true: that if the Savio would pass through Cesena, then I would no longer be a fool."[8]

So these men are the type we call perverted fools, and in our Hospital they have a cell that has the image of the goddess Themis[9] outside. And it is she as their protectress whom we invoke for their sake, with the following oration:

---

[4] Sir Mattio: probably a fool from the Commedia dell'Arte. "Matto" means crazy or deranged in Italian.

[5] "Chopped meat," with the additional meaning of "go to hell."

[6] "I cast my *ballotta* . . . ": a play on *ballotta*, which means both "vote" and "boiled chestnut."

[7] Savignano: on the Rubicon, near Rimini.

[8] A play on the name of the river Savio, and *savio*, meaning wisdom. "If wisdom [*savio*] would flow through Cesena then I would no longer be a fool."

[9] Themis, daughter of Uranus and Ge. In the Homeric epics, she is the personification of the order of things, of laws and customs. She taught Apollo the art of divination: Giraldi, *De deis gentium*, 15 (443).

An Oration to the Goddess Themis on behalf of Perverted Madmen

O Great Daughter of Uranus and Ge, as much loved by Jupiter as you are stingy towards his love, don't be stingy with your help for these souls who, finding themselves insane and perverted, seek from Themis, goddess of Virtuous Requests, that which they need to request. Therefore, they request this rightful and just thing: that you may entreat Uranus, your father, to impart wisdom to their intellects and virtue to their minds. For if, through your grace, they are freed from such an impairment, you will see offered to you, at your temple near the River Cephissus[10] — so greatly honored by the Boeotians — a female Spanish mule which will be a clear sign of the triumph that you suddenly acquire through such a great liberation.

---

[10] Cephissus, ruler of feasts and gatherings; co-planner of the Trojan War; keeper of civic order. Garzoni has "Celiso," but Cephissus is meant. The river Cephissus flows through Boeotia.

The Thirteenth Discourse: The Spiteful and Tarot Types[1]

There are some people who have embedded in their brains such a spirit that, whenever they feel offended or insulted by anyone, they start to do battle with them with an insane willfulness. And just as the insults and offenses multiply from the side of the offender, so also do spiteful acts and hatred grow on their side as well. So it reduces itself to this: that by getting their brains enraged in a beastly manner, they have earned the name of Madmen Spiteful and Full of Wrath.

Perhaps among the ancient examples, the case of Cleomedes of Astypaleia—a man of mighty strength, mentioned by Plutarch—should be placed here.[2] Having been defrauded out of a certain reward due to him because of his prowess, he developed such spite about this thing that one day he went to rest his shoulders against a pillar which supported a school building. All the children of the nobility were there. In a great fury he pushed it to the ground, killing the teacher together with all the children.

In this group we can also place Marganor, whom Ariosto wrote about.[3] Because of the death of his two sons, he held such great rage against the entire female sex that all the women who happened to go through his domain were subjected to cruel pranks and treated wretchedly.

For a great spiteful fool in our times, a certain Latin-spouting braggart[4] has been christened by all. He is like a Belfagor.[5] If he were bitten by a flea, he would

---

[1] Tarot Types: or *tarocco* evokes the playful, trickery of these madmen. Barelli (12 n. 13) suggests that the term connotes "having little value."

[2] Cleomedes was a famous Greek athlete who, frustrated by his failure to win a medal at the Olympic Games of 494, became mad and massacred sixty students and their teachers: Plutarch, *Romulus*, 28. See also Celio, *Lectiones*, 626–27 and Tixier, *Officina*, 2.60. Garzoni also discusses him in his *Teatro*, Discourse 52.

[3] Ariosto, *Orlando Furioso*, 37.

[4] The person whom Garzoni is describing—if he is an historical figure—is unknown.

[5] Thought to have been a divinity worshipped by Moabites near the Dead Sea. In the Middle Ages, he was thought of as a devil and the protagonist of a myth according to which he assumed a human form and married in order to verify that the cause of the fall of man was woman. Machiavelli wrote a *novella* entitled *Belfagor*.

want to massacre the whole world. And when he gets into his nuttiness and onto his crazy wagon, he has no fear of all the artillery of the Duke of Ferrara,[6] because his spite and rancor rob him of all foresight of the dangers and blows that hang over his fury. So, on our theme, it has been reported of him that one day, when someone called him a fiddle-head, he was put into such a rage by this word that he threw such a great punch at the man that, hitting a column, he broke both his hand and his arm. When he realized how much damage he had done to himself, he became even more furious and threw a sack of marble at his forehead. But it hit the wall and ricocheted back and hit him in his stomach. His rage doubled and he tried to butt the man in the stomach with his head. When the man got out of the way, he smashed his head into the wall, crushing it completely. Finally, having no other way to give vent to his rage, he erupted a deep belch saying, "Take this, since I cannot vindicate myself in any other way."

Cristoforo of Crispino was a great spiteful and raging fool. One day, a man said to him (because he was extremely ugly), "You certainly are a lovely boy!" Enraged at this man's ironic speech, he threw a brick of cheese at his stomach. But because the man picked up the cheese and carried it away to eat, he threw a knife at him; but the man took the knife to use it to cut the cheese. And since they were close to a bakery, the fool picked up a loaf of bread and threw it at him. The man picked up the loaves to eat with his cheese. Finally, he meant to throw an empty wine jug that was sitting nearby at him. But the man said to him, "Brother, be so good as to fill it with wine first and then throw it at me!" With these words, the fool became so enraged that he ran to a nearby fountain intending to throw the jug full of water at the man. But the man, laughing and sneaking off like an insidious Parthian,[7] said, "My friend, I will take the knife, the bread, and the cheese: you take the jug of water so that we are even." In this way, he eluded the last blow of the spiteful fool who finally noticed that he was being held in the greatest scorn for his foolish acts.

A more famous example of spiteful madness could not be described than that presented by the divine Ariosto in the perverse and wicked Gabrina, especially in that stanza that begins:

"Listen," she said, "you who are
So mighty, and have such spite and malice for me,
If you knew what news I have of her
Whose death you mourn, what love you'd have for me!

---

[6] The Duke of Ferrara, Alphonso I, had the most powerful artillery on the Italian peninsula in the early sixteenth century.

[7] The Parthians had the reputation of feigning flight so that they could then return and murder their adversaries. They were said to have mastered the art of shooting their arrows behind them while retreating on horseback.

But rather than tell you of her, I'd rather
That you strangle me or chop me into a thousand pieces."[8]

This cursed old wretch, with all her rage and spite, tried to vent her fury at the forlorn Zerbino, showing no sympathy for his fate, without a single scintilla of compassion, like an iniquitous and diabolical witch, which is what she truly was.

These people are therefore deservedly called Madmen Spiteful or Full of Wrath. In our Hospital they have a cell which has the goddess Nemesis[9] out front for a sign. It is to this goddess, in their great need, that we seek recourse, since it is this goddess who commonly takes care of this sort of fool.

An Oration to the Goddess Nemesis on behalf of the Spiteful and Tarot Types

With as much zeal as possible, and with as much vehemence as we are allowed, we plead to you, goddess—called Rhamnusia by the ancients because one can see your image in the Asian city of Rhamnute made by the hand of Pheidias[10]—for your greatest assistance and favor, because we know that there is no better antidote for these spiteful fools than the help of the goddess who, punishing and chastising the lawless and the delinquent, is rightfully considered the healer of these fools' wounds. Therefore, if we obtain that succor which we might well hope for from such a just goddess, know for certain that in thanks for your favors, we will offer up in the temple of Adrastus[11] consecrated to you a basket of garlic and scallions,[12] and everyone will salute the name of Adrastia, spewing forth spiteful odors, clear arguments for the health brought forth to them for whose sake we are addressing the present oration to you. Therefore, heal them, and peace be with you.

---

[8] Ariosto, *Orlando Furioso*, 20.138. In this episode, the evil Gabrina tries to hurt Zerbino by giving him false news of his love, Isabella. The next two lines are, "Now had you been kinder to me, perhaps I would have let you in on my secret."

[9] Goddess of Vengeance. She punished crimes as well as excessive compromising, seeking balance in the affairs of men. She was "the goddess whom none can escape." The Romans considered her to be their "Lady Luck": Giraldi, *De deis gentium* 16. 639–45.

[10] Pheidias may have given up the honor of having created this statue to his student, Agoracritus of Paros.

[11] Adrastus built the first sanctuary to Nemesis on the river Asopus.

[12] *Scalogne*: perhaps a play on *scalogna*, or "bad luck." See also p. 50, note 40, on the Egyptians' worship of garlic and onions.

The Fourteenth Discourse: The Ridiculous

There are some fools who do things all day that are so strange, uncommon, and unusual that, partly because of their novelty and partly because of their excesses, they cause anyone who sees or hears them to laugh. So everybody calls them Ridiculous Fools, giving them the name that conforms to their daily deeds and actions.

The historian Justinus[1] records this one from among the ridiculous follies reported about Sardanapalus, king of the Assyrians: he delighted in womanly adornments beyond measure, so he would sometimes dress himself in women's clothing and join the young girls, handling the bobbin and spindle just as they did, and perform all those activities that women usually do.

Homer's madness also has a place among that of other ridiculous madmen. It has been reported of him that he would have ended his life by miserably strangling himself for this one reason: he could not solve a certain riddle that some sailors or mariners had given to him.[2]

Another fine example is that of the poet Philaemon.[3] As Valerius Maximus[4] has written, when he saw an ass eating some figs placed on a table, he laughed so hard that his sides split.

---

[1] Junianus Justinus Antonius, historian of the age of Anthony, author of an *Epitome* of Trogus' *Historiae Philippicae*. Sardanapalus was considered by the Greeks to be the last king of the Assyrian empire of Nineveh, known for its luxury and sloth. He was very effeminate and sensual and became a symbol of erotic dissoluteness. Ctesias, in his history, states that thirty generations of rulers in Sardanapalus' line were all effeminate. Cf. Tixier, *Officina*, 5.31 (755), and Celio, *Lectiones*, 308. Sardanapalus' story can also be found in Herodotus (*Histories,* 2.150) and Athenaeus (*Deipnosophists,* 12.528).

[2] From Tixier, *Officina,* 2.98. See also M.W. Gahtan, "Giraldi's *Aenigmata,*" in *Acta Conventus Neo-Latini Bonnensis,* ed. R. Schnur et al., MRTS 315 (Tempe: ACMRS, 2006), 315–23.

[3] Philemon (361–262 B.C.), a poet who wrote sixty comedies. The anecdote is in Tixier, *Officina,* 2.88 (230).

[4] Valerius Maximus, *Memorable Doings and Sayings,* 9.12, ext.6; trans. Shackleton Bailey, 2:377.

A similar example is that of Margutte in Luigi Pulci's poem, who burst from laughing when he saw an ape putting on his boots.[5]

Lampridius[6] tells us the following: that among the ridiculous foolishnesses of Elagabalus,[7] he would sometimes ride in a chariot pulled by four naked whores, and sometimes he would visit all of the whorehouses in Rome, handing out wages to all these nasty women whom he termed his chums. Sometimes he would dress up as a whore, letting the whole world know that he was not a Roman emperor but an Imperial Clown.

But the follies of Nero surpass all others,[8] because, wishing to give birth like a woman, he turned himself into both a stallion and a mare at the same time, and with Sporos,[9] his Ganymede, he engaged in this silliness so much that he had the physicians change him from a male into a female.

John Ravisius Tixier[10] included Xenophon among the laughable fools. He was of this nature: the more he tried to keep from laughing, the more intensely he was caught up in laughing.

Athenaeus, in the fifth book of his *Deipnosophists*, where he tells of the foolishness of Antiochus,[11] the mad king of Syria, relates these thoroughly ridiculous stories: he would carry on business and commerce with both the dregs of society and with gentlemen and lords indiscriminately, and he preferred to drink with the viler sorts rather than with nobles. Whenever he learned about any gathering of merry young men, he would join them on the spur of the moment, bringing his zither or lute and mixing with them. Often, putting aside his regal clothing, he went into the streets, lantern in hand, taking this man and that one by the hand, appealing to them to give him their votes and support, because sometimes, in the manner of the Romans, he wanted to be elected aedile and at other times

---

[5] The episode is recounted in Canto XIX, stanza 144 of Luigi Pulci's poem *Morgante* (1480).

[6] Aelius Lampridius, supposedly fourth-century Latin historian, in *Scriptores Historiae Augustae*, trans. D. Magie (Cambridge, MA: Harvard University Press, 1967), 2:162–63, 166–71.

[7] For Elagabalus see *Oxford Classical Dictionary*, 3rd ed. rev. (Oxford: Oxford University Press, 2003), 221–22, 515.

[8] In Tixier, *Officina*, 5.64.

[9] Tixier, *Officina*, 4.86 (604). Sporos was said to bear a striking resemblance to Nero's wife. When she died, Nero had Sporos castrated and dressed as a woman. Nero later married Sporos: Suetonius, *Suetonius, Lives of the Caesars*, "Nero," 28.

[10] Tixier, *Officina*, 7.52 (1049). This is the only time that Garzoni mentions Tixier explicitly even though he supplied the majority of his literary or historical examples. See Introduction.

[11] Antiochus, king of Syria: in Athenaeus, *Deipnosophists*, 5.193 (377ff). Antiochus Epiphanes or "Antiochus the Illustrious" was nicknamed "Antiochus the Insane."

Tribune of the People.[12] Very often, in the presence of noblemen, he would romp around like a buffoon, causing great embarrassment to those who witnessed such a lack of dignity.

Among the ridiculous fools of our own time, we can certainly count the lunatic Pedruccio of Biagrasso, who goes through the streets collecting all the horse and cow dung he can find, and carries it home for ammunition, saying that, in times of need, that crap will be good to make into a pie with which he could save his own life, despite the usurers.[13]

Michelino of Papozze[14] is another sort of half-wit who causes the whole world to laugh because of his foolish acts. In the summertime, he puts a breastplate on his back, a fur coat over it, and then a Roman shield over that, saying that he doesn't want the piercing rays of the sun to penetrate his clothing in any way and make him sweat.

But Santriccio of Ritonda[15] is a ridiculous and mindless fool if there ever was one. All summer he does nothing but catch frogs and skin them. He then takes their skins all together to a furrier to process them, saying that the emperor of Rome never had such a fine and rare fur coat like the one that is about to be fashioned from these frog skins.

All men of this type are therefore called ridiculous fools because they do nutty things that are consistent with the ridiculous ones. Over their cell here in our Hospital, they have the image of the god Risius,[16] adored by the ancients who have dedicated themselves to him as their true god. So with the following ridiculous oration, let us solemnly invoke him for their protection.

An Oration to the God Risus on behalf of the Ridiculous

I cannot—except with uncontrollable bursts of laughter—turn to you, O son of Jupiter, or Bacchus, Friend of All Buffoons, Passionate Lover of Drunkards, Enemy of Boredom even more than of death, nourished by Venus, raised by Cupid, and supported at the goddess Flora's expense, gallant gentleman for life, true merry companion, and, in good times, financial advisor. So on behalf of these

---

[12] aedile: important Roman official, responsible for streets, marketplaces, etc. Tribune of the People: another lofty Roman office with responsibility for protection of the people. Both offices would be well out of reach of this madman.

[13] Pedruccio will throw his lumps of dung at the moneylenders when they come to collect from him.

[14] Papozze, small village on the Po, near Rovigo.

[15] Ritonda, a village now part of the town of San Bonifacio, near Verona.

[16] Personified Laughter, God of the Ridiculous, a divinity more burlesque than mythic, but Giraldi has a place for him in his pantheon of the gods: Giraldi, *De deis gentium,* 55.

men, I cannot help making—with old Democritus[17]—a great squealing laughter just like the kind that Padella[18] makes in the Piazza San Marco. For if it were not for you who help and nurture these ridiculous fools, our whole Hospital would be in a wretched state. Nor would there be anything but sadness and melancholy everywhere. But these men, through your favor, doing their part, certainly keep even the nurses happy and relieve everybody's souls of that sadness produced by the fools afflicted by the frenetic, delirious, melancholic, and savage humors, and by all the others similar to them. Consequently, many people are not a little beholden to you, feeling through you their hearts uplifted and their heartstrings sounding with great joy. So if you persist, as we hope you will with this particular species of fool, be assured that you will hear, in your temple, greater laughter than has ever been heard at the banquets of Elagabalus or of Commodus.[19] All this shall be done to please you who are the cause of all laughter.

---

[17] Democritus, Greek anatomist and philosopher (460–370 B.C.) His moral philosophy led to his being termed "the laughing philosopher," in contrast to the melancholy Heraclitus, "the philosopher who weeps."

[18] Padella: Cherchi suggests that "Padella" should perhaps to be corrected to "Gradella," a character of the Commedia dell'Arte: Cherchi, 302, n. 16.

[19] Commodus (161–192 A.D.), son of Marcus Aurelius, was famous for his bloody despotism. He compromised the work of his father and placed the empire in crisis through his nepotism, corruption, his extravagant spending on festivals, and his delight in banquets. He was said to have had 300 concubines: Tixier, *Officina*, 5.53 (830).

The Fifteenth Discourse: The Vainglorious

The greatest numbers of fools that we can find are probably the ones we will discuss now, making clear and boastful mention of them to the world, and we call them by this boastful term, Boastful Madmen. For they love nothing more, seek nothing more intensely, nor covet anything with greater anxiety, than to be glorified by the world, something that they are more desirous of than the avaricious are of gold, bears are of honey, and bees are of flowers. For this is the meal, the appetizer, and the dessert of all of their actions. And because of this stubborn matter that they have in their heads, they are unable to penetrate with their intelligence the sayings which the wise men have made against them, such as the statement of Aristotle, who, in the books of his secrets, says to Alexander,

Nulla tanta fortitudo est, ut superbiae pondus sustinere valeat.[1]

No strength is powerful enough to sustain the burden of pride.

Or take this by Aristophanes, who said,

Non oportere in civitate nutriri leones.[2]

Don't nurture lions in the city.

Or this one from Demades the Athenian, who, when his fellow citizens wanted to attribute divine honors to Alexander, said,

---

[1] Garzoni is here referring to Pseudo-Aristotle, *Secretum Secretorum*. However, the quotation could not be found there.

[2] From Valerius Maximus, *Memorable Doings and Sayings* 2, ext. 7. Aristophanes, in Aeschylus' *Frogs* (1431f) says, with reference to Alcibiades, "Don't rear a lion in the city, but if one is raised, best do what it wants." Erasmus explains: "He is telling them that young men of exalted birth and lively turn should be reined in, but if fed on overmuch popularity and lavish indulgence they should not be hindered from holding power; for it is foolish and useless to carp at forces which you yourself have encouraged": *Adagia*, 2.3.77 (33: 176–77).

Videt, quaeso, cives, ne, dum ad coelum gloriosum istum tollitis, in terram deiiciatis.[3]

Watch out, good citizens, that while you are praising this man to the heavens, you aren't also throwing him in the dirt.

But they are so blinded by this damned ambition that devours and pierces their hearts that they have lost their wits, their intellect, and whatever enlightenment they had, racing after the least scintilla of this volatile glory, transient as the wind. Their words are perfumed and sweet-smelling like ambergris,[4] nor do their words trip lightly from their tongues without being relished slowly in their mouths like fine sugar. Their movements are made up in the Garden of the Graces to achieve symmetry. Their steps are measured with the instruments of Archimedes; heaven forbid that one is longer than the other or this one shorter than that one. Their bearing is that of a peacock strutting in a barnyard. Their presence is that of a Jove, sitting on his golden throne amidst the gods. Their movement looks like a turtle's, wagging its tail as it walks along the ground.[5] Their pomposity is like that of a goose from Romagna as she moves through the poultry yard. The rolling of their eyes is like that of a cat as it preens itself. When they stand still they are like a toad that seems to focus on the ground. Their speech moves more slowly than an ant when it is carrying more than the usual amount of grain. In sum, all their actions are so affected that you could never find a more irritating or a stranger thing than these boastful fools.

The ancient Arvernians are counted among these boastful fools. As many have reported, they boasted that they were descended from Trojan blood, and for this reason, they called themselves Brothers of the Romans. Lucan wrote of them in his first book:

Arvernique ausi Latios se fingere fratres
sanguine ab iliaco populi.[6]

The Arvernians dared to imagine that they were brothers of the Romans because they had Trojan blood.

---

[3] Valerius Maximus, *Memorable Doings and Sayings*, 7:2, ext. 13 (123). Demades was an Athenian orator and politician under the reign of Alexander. He was noted for his crude eloquence and venality: Fiorato, n. 353. The original statement, made by Demades when the Athenians were unwilling to decree divine honors to Alexander, was, "Take care that in guarding the heavens you don't lose the earth," i.e., "while you are carefully guarding the integrity of the gods, you might lose everything else to Alexander."

[4] Ambergris: the waxy substance secreted by the sperm whale; used in perfume.

[5] Here, Garzoni plays on *Gallone d'India*, the Indian rooster, and *Galana*, a sea turtle.

[6] Lucan, *Pharsalia*, 1.427–428, but also in Tixier, *Officina*, 7.48. The Arvernians were a nation of Celts and, in Caesar's time, one of the most powerful.

Similar to these was a certain Murrano, not the one where goblets[7] are made, but the one that Virgil writes about in the twelfth book of the *Aeneid*:

Murrhanum hic, atavos et avorum antiqua sonantem nomina.

Here comes Murranus, boasting loudly of grandfathers and their grandfathers.[8]

Among other examples of boastful madmen, the ancient writers include Misenus, Aeneas' trumpeter, who considered himself to be so outstanding in his profession that he dared to challenge the sea gods to play the trumpet with him.[9] Similarly, Marsyas provoked the god Apollo into the same sort of contest.[10]

Likewise, the Thracian Tamyras was so audacious that he challenged the Muses to a singing contest. Among these one could also include Arachne, who dared challenge Minerva over wool-weaving. Finally, there is Cassiopeia, daughter of Cepheus,[11] who dared claim superiority to the Nereids; and Niobe to Latona;[12] and Antigone, daughter of Laomedon,[13] to Juno; and Lychion, daughter of Dedalio,[14] to Diana. It is a fact that the tribe of boastful ones is greater than all the others, because in all times it has been proven by experience that the chimney of the brain emits more smoke from this corner than from any other.[15]

What shall we say of Numanus Remulus, who, presuming too much of himself, excessively pleased with his own valor, blamed the Trojans in Italy for being besieged by effeminacy and idleness, since Virgil wrote these words about them:

Is primam ante aciem digna atque indigna relatu
vociferans, tumidusque novo praecordia regno
ibat, et ingentem sese clamore ferebat.

---

[7] Garzoni plays on "Murano," the Venetian town famous for its glassware, and "Murranus" of this anecdote. The story is told in *Aeneid*, 12.529–530.

[8] All of these examples of mythical contests between presumptuous fools and the gods are found in Tixier, *Officina*, 5.24 (741–43), *On Arrogance, Pride, and Ambition*.

[9] Virgil, *Aeneid*, 3.239.

[10] Marsyas' punishment for losing his musical contest with Apollo was to be skinned alive.

[11] Cassiopeia was actually Cepheus' wife. According to one account, because she boasted that she was more beautiful than the Nereids, she was punished by being chained to her throne and placed in the sky to circle the North Star. Half the time she is right-side up, and half upside down.

[12] Niobe claimed to be more blessed with children than Latona, who retaliated by having Artemis kill all of Niobe's girls, and Apollo kill all of her boys: Apollodorus, 3:5, 7.

[13] For her arrogance, Juno turned Antigone into a crane: Ovid, *Metamorphoses*, 5.93 f.

[14] Garzoni has "Deucalione" here.

[15] See p. 41, note 5.

Now this captain strode ahead and shouted
Boasts that had or had not dignity,
Inflated as he was by his new status.[16]

And what can we say of Mariccus,[17] one of the vilest riffraff among the Boians, who, according to Cornelius Tacitus, dared to declare himself a god? And what of Apion the grammarian, who would promise certain immortality to anyone to whom he dedicated one of his works?[18] And boastful beyond measure was Menecrates, the physician, who usually expected no payment for freeing his patients from disease, but asked only this: that they call themselves his servants and consider him another Jove.[19]

The heretic Nestorius[20] was also one of them, because in one of his orations made to the people of Constantinople he so pleased himself that the next day he promised to grant heaven to every one of them.

And Rhemnius Palaemon,[21] the grammarian and pedant, is not so far off from these, because he usually boasted about himself that *belles lettres* had been born with him and would die with him.

And why leave out Paul of Samosata,[22] who went through the squares, streets, and alleys ostentatiously making public his ideas and had certain scribes write down everything that came, *ipso facto*, from his mouth? And why do I pass in silence over the Emperor Domitian, who pleased himself with nothing as much as this: to be called Lord and God? So Eusebius wrote:

---

[16] Garzoni refers to this quotation in his *Theater*, Discourse 42, note 42; *Aeneid*, 9. 595–597. The "new status" is an allusion to the recent marriage of Remulus Numanus to Turnus' daughter. The young Ascanius killed the insolent Latin with an arrow.

[17] Mariccus was a Gaul who incited the peasants to revolt agains Vitellus. Tacitus (*Histories*, trans. Morre, 2.61) explains that once he was captured and "exposed to the beasts . . . the animals did not rend him, [so] the stupid rabble believed him inviolable, until he was executed before the eyes of Vitellus."

[18] Apion is mentioned in Josephus' *Contra Apionem* as his antagonist (2. 13).

[19] Menecrates, physician to Philip of Macedon. He wrote to Philip: "You are king of Macedon; I am king of Medicine." Philip once invited him to dinner and fed him only libations and incense — since Menecrates considered himself a god. He was not amused and left: Athenaeus, *Deipnosophists*, 7.289 (3: 297, 299).

[20] Nestorius vowed to Theodosius II that if he would "free (the land) of heretics . . . I will give you heaven in return": see Timothy E. Gregory, *Vox Populi: Popular Opinion and Violence in the Religious Controversies of the Fifth Century A.D.* (Columbus, OH: Ohio State University Press, 1986), 84.

[21] Quintus Remnius Palaemon, Roman grammarian, lived in the reigns of Tiberius and Claudius. He was insufferably arrogant, but also considered a great teacher. Quintilian and Galen may have been his students.

[22] Paul of Samosata: Bishop of Antioch; he was accused of heresy c. 264. See *Oxford Dictionary of the Christian Church*, 3rd ed. (Oxford: Oxford University Press, 1997), 1242.

Primus Domitianus se dominum et deum appellari iussit.

Domitian was the first to command that he would be called Lord and God.²³

So a certain poet, a flatterer of his, wrote these two lines:

Edictum domini deique nostri,
quo subsellia certiora fiunt.

The edict of our Lord and God,
Whereby the benches are more stictly assigned.²⁴

And why would I leave out Caius Princeps,²⁵ who produced an edict that he be numbered among the gods and that statues should be erected to him with the name Greatest Caesar? Nor will I forget Themison of Cyprus,²⁶ who made people call him Hercules and praise him and make him illustrious through divine prayers like that god.

What shall we say of Nero, who, desiring eternal fame, had the month of April renamed Neroneus, and, according to Suetonius, decided that Rome should be called Neropolis?²⁷

Alexander of Macedon, for his part, can also be placed among these boastful fools because he gained extreme pleasure from being called the son of Jupiter Ammon.²⁸

---

²³ Tixier, *Officina*, 5.24. The story was not found in Eusebius, *Ecclesiastical History* but in Eutropius, *Abridgment of Roman History* 7.23 (trans. John Selby Watson [London: Henry G. Bohn, 1853]), 506. Tacitus, *History* 3.74 reports that Domitian also dedicated "a great temple to Jupiter the Guardian with his own effigy in the lap of the god."

²⁴ Martial, *Epigrams* 5.8, also in Tixier, *Officina* 5.24 (745). Martial is speaking about how Domitian (A.D. 81–96)—"Our Lord and God"—would assign theater seats to the noblemen.

²⁵ Caius Princeps: Caligula. Suetonius (*Lives of the Twelve Caesars: Caligula*) termed Caius a "monster."

²⁶ Antiochus II, king of Syria would dress Themison as Hercules and order the people to make sacrifices to him. Athenaeus, *Deipnosophists*, 7: 289; 10: 438; Aelian, *Historia varia* 2:41.

²⁷ Suetonius (9 [2:177]) reports that Nero "had a longing for immortality and undying fame, though it was ill-regulated."

²⁸ Quintius Curtius Rufus (*History of Alexander* 4.7.5–30) reports this remarkable story. Jupiter Ammon frequently visited Philip's wife, Olympias, appearing in the form of a snake. Philip discovered that Alexander was in reality the son of Jupiter Ammon because he watched—through a keyhole—Olympias and Jupiter having intercourse. Philip was punished by Jupiter by causing him to lose the eye with which he had seen the lovers.

Salmoneus imitated the sounds of thunder and lightning by using the discipline of mathematics for no other purpose than to acquire the fame of a god.[29]

Varrus of Perge, corrupted by the words of yes-men, easily became convinced that he was the most handsome man among all of the men in the world and that he could sing more sweetly and divinely than the Muses.

Hanno the Carthaginian frequently caught birds and taught them to say the phrase: "Hanno is god."[30]

Sellus was certainly a poor braggart, since he used to hide his own poverty as much as he could, because he longingly desired the praise of the whole world for being thought of as wealthy.

According to Aulus Gellius, Herostratus, that truly vainglorious fool, burned down the temple of Diana at Ephesus solely to achieve immortal fame in the world.[31]

Finally, Empedocles of Agrigentum,[32] a crazy above all other crazies, threw himself into the flames of Mount Aetna so that people would think that he had, without a doubt, flown up to heaven.

In our times, the number of these boastful fools has increased so much that there is no place so small that one cannot find an immense crowd of them there. The example of that Tuscan as boastful as Thraso[33] is truly a very special one in our era: he was asked by some good friends why, on a certain occasion, he had not got into a fight. He replied that the reason was as follows: he knew that his hands were so massive and heavy that if he used them he would instantly kill someone.

No less pleasing is the story of Valentino from Castel San Piero[34] who, having been slapped by an innkeeper in the public square, went away with bravado and laughter, saying these words: "That guy turned to me and slapped me because he didn't have enough guts to punch me with his fist, because had he punched me like that, woe to him! I would have poked him in the nose with another blow that would have destroyed him!"

Alexander spoke of his father as Jupiter Ammon. He verified the paternity by visiting the oracle of Jupiter Ammon at Siwa (Egypt) and being hailed as the god's son.

[29] See R.S. Smith and S.M. Trzaskoma, "Apollodorus 1.9.7: Salmoneus' Thunder-Machine," *Philologus*, 149 (2005): 351–54.

[30] In Aelian, *Historia varia*, 14. 30 (trans. Johnson, 332–33).

[31] In fact, Aulus Gellius did not name Herostratus as the perpetrator of this deed, since he considered him to be *inlaudabilis*, or one who is unworthy of mention or remembrance: *Attic Nights* 2:18.

[32] Empedocles of Agrigentum, fl. 444 B.C.: Diogenes Laertius, *Lives* 8.74.

[33] Thraso: boastful soldier in Terence's *Eunuch*.

[34] Castel San Piero: today Castel San Pietro Terme, 20 miles southeast of Bologna on the Via Emilia.

Fools of this type have their own cell in our Hospital. Outside it features the image of Juno to whom they are naturally commended and whom I solemnly implore on behalf of them with the oration that follows:

An Oration to the Goddess Juno on Behalf of the Vainglorious

O greatest Goddess of Goddesses, Queen of Heaven,[35] Spouse and Sister of great Jupiter, most glorious among all the gods—just as the sun is the most glorious among all the planets—I pray that you take care of these boastful fools, since this seems to befit your deity. Again I pray to you with these glorious epithets: Saturnia, because you are the daughter of Saturn; Aeria, because you rule over air; goddess Curetis, because you ride in a chariot with a spear in your hand; Lucina and Lucetia, because you give light to all who are about to be born; Socigena, because you join males and females in matrimony; Iuga,[36] Populonia, Domiduca, Interduca, and Unxia. May these fools be commended to you and may they be defended and saved under the shadow of your wings.

And you are also Opigena, Helper of Pregnant Women, and Februa, or Februata, who, via the monthly flow, purges the female sex; and Fluonia who has the power to coagulate the menstrual blood when women conceive. Therefore, just as you provide all these various helps, so help these fools too.

May you be completely helpful to them with your name so that, in addition to the temple that you have on the Lacinian promontory (so you are called Lacinia); and in addition to your chapel in the Argivian town of Prosymnos (so you are called Prosymna); and in addition to the altar which the Etruscans built for you in the Marquisate of Ancona (so you are called Cupra);[37] may you also see a temple erected in our Hospital because of which you will be called Hospitalaria, just as your husband is called Jupiter Hospital. Then may everyone add to your titles Pelasga, Goddess Moneta, Goddess Castrensis,[38] Goddess Caprotina, Goddess Sospita, and Goddess Calendare—yet another title, Boastful, because you provided much-needed succor for such an enormous squadron of boastful fools, who vow, because of your

---

[35] For Juno's epithets, see Giraldi, *De deis gentium*, 3, 117-30.

[36] The text has "Iuga," however, Cherchi (307, n. 22) believes that it should read "Fuga."

[37] Cupra or Cypra, today called Cupramarittima, where one can still see the remains of the ancient temple.

[38] Castrensis: not listed in Giraldi. It is also an epithet of the Roman goddess, Bona Dea, with whom Juno is sometimes identified. See Hendrick Brouwer, *Bona dea: The Sources and Description of the Cult* (Utrecht: University of Utrecht, 1982) 299.

great assistance, to erect a tower to you—higher than the one at Cremona[39]—where torches will be lit so that the whole world will know of the glory of Juno, who is made more glorious by this one single act than by all of her previous ones.

---

[39] Built between 1267 and 1305, the clock tower in Cremona, at 110 meters, is the tallest in Europe.

The Sixteenth Discourse:
The Fakers and Jokers

It is not such an obvious matter that these fools that we term Fakers or Joking Fools should have a place in our Hospital for Incurable Madness, since they are not really fools in the sense that the others are, and therefore have little in common with this collection,[1] but, on the contrary, it seems more appropriate to place them with the sages, since as Cato, that wise man, said:

Stultitiam simulare loco, prudentia summa est.

It is sometimes wise to wear the fool's mask.[2]

So we attribute great wisdom to the astrologer Meson,[3] who, foreseeing the future calamity about to befall his countrymen, the Athenians, in their expedition against the Sicilians, feigned madness so that he would not be with them to witness their undoing.

Similarly, we read of the prudent Ulysses,[4] who, in order not to go to the Trojan war, sowed salt like a fool, and, hitching together various and sundry animals to his plow, amazed everyone with his sudden madness. Only Palamedes discovered his ruse by putting his baby boy in the furrows; when the wary Greek wisely avoided him, he clearly demonstrated, by that act, that he was in control of his faculties and not at all crazy.

But because there are undoubtedly some people who at times play the fool as a joke, using a touch of folly that they have in their heads — it being a sign of

---

[1] Garzoni here touches upon a widely-discussed theme of the sixteenth century: the wisdom of fools. For example, Erasmus, *Adagia*, 1.14.91, "*Nugas agene*," "to play the fool" (31: 378). See the Introduction, p. 1ff.

[2] *Disticha Catonis*, 2.18.2; Cherchi, 308, n. 1.

[3] Meson or Methon: his prophecy is mentioned in Agrippa, *Three Books of Occult Philosophy*, 3.64 (673). His feigned madness is reported in Aelian, *Historia varia*, 13.12. Tixier, *Officina* 4:19 (448), where he is referred to as Alcibiades Metheon. He was an Athenian astronomer of the fifth century B.C. Fiorato (n. 382) reports that he was the inventor of the "golden number."

[4] In Tixier, *Officina*, 2:60 (214). This story is not in Homer, but rather the *Cypria*. See Apollodorus, *Epitome*, 3.7; Pliny, *Natural History*, 35.129; Hyginus, *Fabulae*, 95.

madness to play the fool for no other reason than to amuse others—it is only to these that we are referring when we put these Fakers and Joker Madmen into our Hospital.

There is certainly no doubt that we can place Gallus Vibius[5] among these men. Noted by Celio in the thirty-fifth chapter of the sixth book of his *Ancient Lectures*, he would frequently fake being mad and, joking like this, in the end he completely lost his mind so that, whereas he previously had made fun of other people, he ended up being the brunt of other people's jokes as a punishment for his foolishness.

In our times, Garbinello[6] is known for the charming way he plays the madman, just as he has no equal when playing a Paduan peasant, or a Magnifico, or a Graziano, so in this other type of dissimulation he surpasses all others, because anyone who sees him or hears his voice, seeing his movements, gestures, and words, would be certain that he was indeed a fool.

Pedretto of Moiano[7] proved himself to be his worthy competitor. When the Venetian lords, because of some special need, forced ordinary servants to work on the galley ships, they commanded him to go too, but he, like many others, avoided being a galley-slave. But to give some pleasure to certain gentlemen friends of his with whom he had made a deal, he showed up one day before the captain of this gang of galley rowers dressed as a galley-slave, with a chain around his ankle. And, with oar in hand, he began to row all by himself for a little while. Then, taking the pipe that is used on these galleys, he blew the most beautiful call that could ever be imagined. Then, having a sackful of biscuits with him, he began to distribute pieces of biscuit among the crew. He also took a big piece to the captain, telling him that these, together with a head of garlic, would make a fabulous meal. Finally, he picked up a Turkish scimitar and, unsheathing it in the midst of the crew, he began to cry out, "*Allai, allai maumeth russelai.*"[8] He began to make slashing thrusts at the wind, first here, then there, until finally, all sweaty and exhausted, with everyone watching him, he threw himself to the ground as if he were dead. Then, wrapping himself in a sailor's blanket, he called for a notary to take down his last will and testament. Then, bequeathing something to this one and something else to another, he said that he was bequeathing to the Captain

---

[5] In Tixier, *Officina*, 2.60 where he cites Celio, *Lectiones*, 6.13.

[6] Probably one of the actors in the Commedia dell'Arte who could play a wide variety of roles, including a villain from Padua, who personifies ignorance; a Magnifico, a pretentious aristocrat; and a Dr. Graziano, representing absurd science. Dr. Graziano would conclude a scholarly-sounding speech by stating, "He who is wrong cannot be right," or "A Ferrarese cannot be a Mantuan," or "One who is asleep cannot be said to be awake."

[7] Moiano: perhaps the small town four miles south of Lake Trasimeno.

[8] A garbled version of the Arabic "There is no god but Allah [and] Mohammed is his prophet."

of the Rabble a great rascal and a great rogue to bury. And since he was a galley-slave, he wished to be buried in no other place than the galley's bilge, because that was the place that was most compatible with his knavery. Then he feigned being dead and they wanted to carry him off, but he suddenly jumped up laughing and said to the Captain, "Signor Captain, I can assure you that among all of these galley-slaves that you have drafted, there is not one who is as god-forsaken as I am, so release me now, for mercy's sake, because if you don't, your galley will be known as the most god-forsaken galley of Venice." So the captain, laughing and taking great delight in the entertainment, contented himself to let him go this time because he had played the fool so marvelously. And, in addition, giving him a *mocenigo*,[9] he said, "Pray to God that even though you have escaped the galley this time that you may not end up on the gallows next time."

Now, these are the madmen who, in front of their cell in our Hospital, display the insignia of Mercury, the god of rogues and criminals like themselves. To him I direct the following oration, praying for the protection of people like this.

An Oration to the God Mercury,[10] on Behalf of Fakers and Jokers

Whatever benefit one could hope for from the son of Jupiter and Cyllene[11] is to be expected from you regarding these fools, O Great Interpreter of the Gods, because these sorts are ones who truly conform themselves so completely to your genius that they seem to all the world like your brothers.

As you can see, these are fakers, and you are the god of deception, since it was you who, with such exquisite deceit, stole Apollo's cattle from Argo, his herdsman. But if this is not enough to earn you the famous epithets which you have obtained from the poets—first, Hermes, or interpreter of words; then Camillus, or minister, since you are the messenger of the mighty Jove; then Alipedis, because of the wings that you have on your sides[12] as the heavenly messenger; then Maiugena, because you were born of Maia, daughter of Atlas; then Arcadian, because you were born in Arcadia; then Cyllenius because you were born on Mount Cyllene; then Logios,[13] Agriphon, and Nomius; all with fervent prayers beseech you to take such care of them as befits such a great god, and as they believe is appropriate to their warm entreaties. And to spur you on even more

---

[9] Venetian currency named for a prominent family.
[10] For Mercury's epithets, see Giraldi, *De deis gentium*, 295–309.
[11] Mercury was the son of Zeus and Maia, as Garzoni correctly points out a few lines later. He was born in a cave on Mount Cyllene in Arcadia (*Odyssey* 8.335).
[12] Although Mercury is usually depicted as having wings on his feet, Garzoni has them attached to his *fianchi* or flanks.
[13] The text has "Ligio," another example of Garzoni's mutilation of epithets.

in this endeavor, they are putting before your eyes many of the honorable acts you have done, such as inventing the lyre, wrestling, commerce, and rhetoric; teaching the Egyptians to write, freeing Mars from prison, binding Prometheus to Mount Caucasus and causing him to be torn to pieces by falcons. They pray to you to add to such illustrious past deeds a deliberate and powerful defense of this species of madman. And if you help them, you can expect that, without a doubt, they will place a fox's pelt[14] before your image in the Temple of the Phoenicians, a gift appropriate to both you and them.

---

[14] The fox is the emblematic deceiver. See Theobald, *Bestiary* (London: Bumpus, 1928), 72. Also Aesop, *Fables,* "The Fox and the Crow."

The Seventeenth Discourse:
The Lunatics or Episodic Crazies

There are very few people who do not know this type of fool only by their name, the ones we call Lunatics or Episodic Crazies who, because they are not constantly vexed by this frenzy, but only occasionally and at certain periods of time, they have been given the name of lunatics since they show mutability in their mental illness, just like the moon; or, rather, because this kind of madness is characteristic and common to those born in the inter-lunal period; or because, just as the moon waxes and wanes according to its various states, this sickness becomes excessive at times and at other times its power is markedly attenuated.

For this reason Julius Firmicus says, in the fourth book of his *Mathematics*,

Et si luna male fuerit collocata, aut spasticos, aut lunaticos, aut caducos facit.[1]

If the moon is in an unfavorable aspect, it produces either spastics, lunatics, or epileptics.

On this topic, I may produce the examples of Nicoletto of Francolino,[2] and Lorenzino[3] of Chioggia. The first one, only when the moon was new, would sometimes get into such a humor that he believed that he had become a shrimp, so he sought out all of the waters in the area in order to take shelter in them. At other times he believed he had turned into a snail, and would put a couple of horns on his head to imitate its nature. At still other times he would be a leek or a clove of garlic, running among the greengrocers crying out, "Who will buy some fine vegetables?" At other times he had turned into sausage or prosciutto and would steer clear of the lard-renderers more than he would if they had been Death itself, fearing that they would chop him up.

The second one, at the waning of the moon, had a waning of wits as well, so that he would run naked through the *piazza* displaying all his private parts. At other times, enveloped in a large wicker basket, he would go through the

---

[1] *Matheseos libri VIII*, 4.5. Julius Firmicus Maternus, Roman astronomer of the fourth century, author of eight books of astronomy: Fiorato, n. 405.

[2] Francolino: on the Po a few miles north of Ferrara.

[3] Lorenzino: in Cherchi, it is "Lorenzo."

square bumping into anyone he happened to meet. But at other times, becoming completely scatter-brained, he would hit people with sticks and stones. Sometimes—and this was something unusually laughable—in the middle of the *piazza* he would flagellate himself on his naked buttocks with the intestine of an ox and then run after the boys with the filthy rotten intestines, throwing them at those who came close to him, just as small birds flock around an owl.[4]

Sandrino of Pietra Mala[5] was also a lunatic and, suffering from this indisposition of the brain, one day, when the moon was full, he did crazy things that are most ridiculous to hear about. Among many, this one is told: he found a certain tavern or road-house which had displayed outside a crown of laurels as its sign. He put this crown on his head and began to say that he was a poet, and began to sing anything that came to his mind. A circle of people gathered around him and, when he saw a whore who happened to be named Diana while he was obsessed by that frenzy,[6] he sang these verses about her:

Look at that Arabian mare,
The one who calls herself Diana:
Diana Ugly, Filthy, Stained, Disgusting,
She's a monkey, baboon, she-goat, sow.

Then, spying a certain pedant in another spot, he sang these verses about him:

Domine qui rudibus insignas pervertere leges,
Tu semper Corydon atque Menalcas eris.[7]

O sir, you who teach the uneducated to pervert the laws,
You will always be a Corydon and a Menalcas.[8]

Among these lunatics we may also place Menegone of Olmo. When the moon was waning, his brain went that way too, and he would go picking up chicory in the ditches. And he would frequently bring bundles of nettles and wild thistles to market, aiming to sell these miserable weeds in place of the chicory. Sometimes he would go fishing for frogs and would fill a tray full of toads instead because he didn't know the difference. Still other times, he would play the tin-plater, and would go through the towns, all black as coal, crying, "Who needs their pans

---

[4] A play on "civetta," meaning "little owl," and "civettone," meaning "fop." See p. 194, notes 19 and 20.

[5] Pietra Mala is a town in the Tuscan Apennines.

[6] A spoof on the idea of "poetic frenzy," a popular concept among sixteenth-century Neo-Platonists.

[7] Sandrino's Latin grammar leaves much to be desired.

[8] Corydon and Menalcas: shepherds in Virgil's *Eclogues* 2 and 3, depicted as homosexuals.

or tin cups or candlesticks or Madonnas fixed?" The only things about him that had anything to do with being a tin-plater were the smoke and the color of his moustache and the filthy sack he carried over his shoulder—all done for the effect they gave.

So this is the type of lunatic that we have spoken about. Over the door to their cell in our Hospital they have hung the sign of Hecate,[9] who is their favorite and, according to our usual practice, the one to whom we address the following oration:

An Oration to the Goddess Hecate on Behalf of Lunatics and Episodic Crazies

Be always blessed and filled with infinite praise—Gentle Daughter of Latona,[10] sister of the god Apollo, deservedly named Hecate because for you the unburied must wander about for one hundred years,[11] just as these poor fools, whom we call lunatics, wander about in their heads. O Triform Goddess,[12] may you happily bestow your gentle influences on this sick rabble because they, with great anxiety, are constantly hoping for it from you. Succor, I pray you, this your feeble, wandering flock, for as soon as your assistance for such dear friends appears to be at hand, there will also immediately appear in your honor in three solemn temples that you have—one in the city of Perge in Pamphylia, another in Ephesus, and the third in the region of Taurus—a memorial trophy of three Turkish flags with the Ottoman's sign in the middle.[13] They will clearly indicate to everyone the good which you have done for them and the disease which has been lifted and removed from them by your grace.

---

[9] Hecate: Lunar goddess of the night and of magic. For her attributes and epithets, Garzoni follows Giraldi, *De deis gentium*, 12 (356–82).

[10] Ovid, *Metamorphoses*, 7.74, describes her as the sister of Latona.

[11] "deservedly named" because her name is derived from the Greek "hecaton," or "one hundred": Giraldi, *De deis gentium*, 359.

[12] Hecate is also the Triform Goddess, since she also incorporates two other goddesses, Diana and Luna: Ovid, *Metamorphoses*, 7.94.

[13] The Turkish flag displayed a crescent moon. The places mentioned were all under Ottoman Turkish rule.

The Eighteenth Discourse: The Love-Mad

Now it would be necessary to have the knowledge and experience of all the cases of love that ever were, in both ancient times and modern ones, in order to describe with appropriate gravity all the madnesses of lovers. They are the obvious cause of a thousand other types of folly which, drawing their being from this source as from their principle and origin, make their lives not only seem to be, but truly to be, the most insane that one could possibly imagine.

This madness seems to be principally rooted in thoughts, desires, ideas, resolutions, words, gestures, signs, and actions. All of these things acting together make a man foolish in matters of love to such an extreme that this material surpasses any other material that I have written about so far.

With foolish thoughts the insane lover creates his own castles in the air, all day fantasizing about what the shortest and fastest way is to implement his lascivious thoughts, which make him restless, troubled, afflicted, and passionate around the clock. So he thinks about treasures, riches, states, dominions, power, and empires as the quickest ways to conquer his beloved object. Together with these thoughts, he mixes in longings for the riches of Croesus, for Midas' gold, for the power of Caesar, and for the comforts of Commodus.[1] Then he considers using incantations, sorceries, charms, and all sorts of magical spells, wishing to make himself invisible with the jewel of Gyges,[2] or with heliotrope. He tries

---

[1] Proverbial examples. For the extravagant enjoyment of pleasure by Commodus, see also p. 112, note 17.

[2] Fiorato, n. 425 corrects this reference to the "ring of Gygis" or Gyges. He was king of Lydia in the seventh century B.C. (Herodotus, *Histories*, 1.7–12). Erasmus's adage suggests that having the "ring of Gyges" refers to those who are truly lucky. Gyges used his ring to become invisible and seduce the king's wife and then conspire with her to kill the king and take his throne: Erasmus, *Adages*, 1.1.96 (31: 138–39) and Manuzio, *Adages* (71–72). Both this ring and the heliotrope (here the stone, not the plant) were two magical substances which could render someone invisible. In his *Theater*, Discourse 15, Garzoni discusses the madness of lovers. Tixier discusses Gyges briefly, *Officina*, 2.24 (123).

to promise the secrets of Pietro d'Abano[3] or those of Ciecco d'Ascoli[4] or those of Antonio de Fantis;[5] or to know how to use Solomon's keys,[6] and to conjure up the power of demons. On the one hand, he considers using alchemy to make himself rich by giving him silver and gold,[7] and make him attain the object of his love. On the other hand, he ponders fallacious Cabalism which, by virtue of mysterious names, might cause his lady to do what he wishes. In this way, he expands his thoughts in a thousand directions: toward finding pimps, procuresses, servants, religious bigots, wet-nurses, chambermaids; toward writing letters, little notes, sonnets, madrigals, or songs; toward sending flowers, bouquets, presents, rewards, and gifts; toward fashioning for himself his miserable amorous servitude using words of great feeling. Little by little he loses his mind, and wears out his wit and intelligence with these fantasies. Burning with these silly longings, he wishes to be a flea or a fly or even an ant so that he can enter his beloved's chambers. He wishes he could make underground tunnels just as rabbits do to accomplish the same goal. He hungers after all sorts of greatness, of beauty, of gifts, of grace, of knowledge beyond anything in the world, in order to obtain her grace. And, what is worse, he wishes that both death and life would come to him at the same instant.[8] In his mind, he creates amorous deeds, elegant and pretty witticisms, sweet and gentle verses, sententious pronouncements, artful sayings, polished ruses. He constructs in his soul, day and night, whatever he thinks will provide him some advantage towards his goal. With his decisions, he plans to put an end to it and be steadfast in his resolve, deciding within himself not to remain like this any more, wanting to stop suffering from further anxiety, and to stop bearing any more torment and paying attention to what she says . But look at what he says and what he thinks and what he resolves with his words! He confronts her and speaks with her, sometimes bitterly, sometimes sweetly, sometimes with an in-between flavor. With his gestures he moves her to compassion, forming his arms into a cross, and he makes her pine away with pity, when he knows how to use his words and actions. In sum, he comports himself in such a way that beasts are sometimes more wise and more prudent than one of the love-mad.

---

[3] Pietro d'Abano (1257–1315), physician and Averroist, astronomer and astrologer. He taught at the University of Paris and was condemned by the church in 1315.

[4] Ciecco (or Cecco) d'Ascoli was a physician, astronomer, and poet, and author of the allegorical poem *Acerba*. He was executed for heresy in 1317.

[5] Antonio de Fantis (end of fifteenth century-early sixteenth century) was the author of works on ancient philosophy and on Duns Scotus, and was the editor of the *Astrorum scientia* of Abd al-Aziz al-Kabisi.

[6] The *Keys of Solomon,* a popular sixteenth-century work on magic arbitrarily attributed to the biblical king.

[7] An allusion to the Philosopher's Stone, the means by which lead could be changed into gold.

[8] The classical Petrarchan conceit, here ridiculed by Garzoni.

A rare example of love-madness was the Roman Mark Antony. Because he was madly in love with Cleopatra, Queen of Egypt, he lost his power, his life, and his honor solely for her.[9]

Nor can we pass over in silence the madness of Pyramus and Thisbe who died miserably—each for the other. So Strozza the Elder describes their death in the following verses:

> *Pyramus exemplum praebet, miserandaque Thisbe,*
> *Quos rapuit simili mors violenta modo.*

Pyramus and the miserable Thisbe offer an example of it:
One violent death took them both in the same way.[10]

And Calentius, in his *Epigrams*, writes this about them:

> *Pyramus et Thisbe miseri sine crimine amarunt,*
> *Occidit hic propria saevus uterque manu.*

Pyramus and Thysbe, miserable ones, loved without fault
And both died cruelly by their own hands.[11]

A very famous example is that of Hercules who was madly in love with Omphale, Queen of Lydia, and because of his love for her, he dressed up as a girl and took to spinning like women among the young maidens. So Propertius put it in this way:

> *Idem ego sydonia feci servilia palla,*
> *Officia et Lydo pensa diurna colo;*

---

[9] Garzoni follows the common tradition of attributing Mark Antony's defeat to his being overly consumed with love for Cleopatra. He follows Tixier, *Officina* 2.98 (270). Fiorato (n. 435) points out that Antony had made a political decision to expand his empire to the East, contrary to the interests of Rome.

[10] Like Romeo and Juliet, Pyramus and Thisbe were lovers forbidden by their parents to marry. They ran away together, but, like Shakespeare's star-crossed lovers, they ended up killing themselves. Fiorato (n. 437) points out that rather than cite the ancient source for this story, Ovid's *Metamorphoses*, Garzoni choses two sixteenth-century writers as his sources. "Strozza the Elder" is the Ferrarese poet Vespasiano Strozzi (1424–1505). The quotation comes from his elegy "De discessu Anthiae ex urbe Ferrariae," verses 23–24, in *Eroticon*, 1, 22–23. His son Ercole was also a poet. Their work was published by Aldo Manuzio: *Strozzi poetae, pater et filius* (Venetiis: Aldi et A. Asulani soceri, 1513). But Garzoni's more likely source is Tixier, *Officina*, 2.98 (278), where one finds the verses cited above from Calenzio and Strozzi: Cherchi, 315, n. 5.

[11] In *Epigrammata*, I, epitaph *"Huc agite ignari"* by the late-fifteenth-century Neapolitan poet Luigi Galluccio, called Calenzio or Calentius, as in Tixier, *Officina*, 2.98 (254): Fiorato, n. 437.

Mollis et hirsutum caepit mihi fascia pectus,
Et manibus duris apta puella fui.

I have also performed menial service dressed in a Sidonian gown
And completed my daily stint at the Lydian distaff;
A soft breast-plate once confined my shaggy chest,
And for all my rough hands, I proved a likely girl.[12]

Similarly, the case of Haemon of Thebes is a notable example; he killed himself in front of the tomb of Antigone, daughter of Oedipus and Jocasta, because of his love for her.[13] And so did Sappho, who threw herself from the Leucadian promontory because of Phaon. Angelo Poliziano, in his *Elegies*, wrote this about her:

Mascula quaeque suos cantat moritura calores
Leucadii Sappho crimen honorque freti.

The courageous Sappho who, dying, sings of her loves;
She was the glory and the shame of the Leucadian sea.[14]

Phaedra hanged herself for her love of Hippolytus. Ausonius said this about her:

Suasi quod potui, tu alios modo consule. Dic quos,
Phaedra et Elisa tibi dent laqueum, aut gladium.

I have advised you as much as I can; now you reflect and tell me what other means there are.
Phaedra and Elisa will give you either the noose or the sword.[15]

---

[12] Propertius, *Elegies*, 4.9.47–50. All of these examples are in Tixier, *Officina*, 2.98, 1.22, 2.32, and 5.35.

[13] The suicide of Haemon, son of Creon and lover of Antigone, ended the tragic Theban story with a double catastrophe: Fiorato, n. 441. According to one account, Haemon killed himself when he heard that Antigone had been condemned by her father to be entombed alive.

[14] The attribution of this story to Poliziano's *Elegies* is incorrect. The story is in Tixier, *Officina*, 2.98 (257), where the quote is attributed to "Bapt. Pius," probably Blessed Baptista Mantuanus.

[15] Cf. Ausonius, *Epigrammata*, 23. 11–12 (trans. Evelyn White, 2:167). Tixier, *Officina* 2.98 (257), where one also finds the reference to Ausonius. The lines in Ausonius are s,omewhat different. There, in a dialogue between Venus and Hippolytus, he, "a poor lover," is asking her for advice on what he should do about being in love. Venus' final advice, if all else fails, is to kill himself like Phaedra and Elisa did. Elisa (or Elissa or Elissar), Queen of Carthage, was Virgil's model for Dido.

Then there is Dido, who threw herself into the roaring fire for her love of Aeneas. So Silius Italicus wrote:

Ipsa pyram super ingentem stans saucia Dido
Mandabat Tyriis ultrici bella futuris
Ardentemque rogum media spectabat ab unda
Dardanus, et magnis pandebat carbasa fatis.

Then Dido by herself was standing on a huge pyre
And charging a later generation of Tyrians to avenge her by war;
And the Dardan, out at sea, was watching the blazing pile
And spreading his sails for his high destiny.[16]

Phyllis, daughter of Lycurgus, King of Thrace, provided a notable example: she hanged herself from a rafter because of her love of Demophoon, son of Theseus. Her death is described by Pamphilus Saxus in these verses:

Exemplum tribuit mortis mihi nobile Phillis
  Pendebat longa corpus inane trave.

For me, Phyllis provides a noble example of death:
Her body hung lifeless from a long beam.[17]

Was not Aristotle's madness great, since he offered incense to one of his concubines as if she were a goddess?[18] And Nero's too, who married Sporos, a boy, and Doriplorus, his freed slave? Or that of Periander[19] the Corinthian who, according to Herodotus, had intercourse with the whore Melissa after she had died?[20] And isn't the love of Semiramis a most powerful example?[21] According to Celio in his thirty-seventh book and according to Justin in his first, she became madly enamored of a bull.[22]

---

[16] Silius Italicus, *Punica*, 2:422 (trans. Duff, 1:90–91). .

[17] Pamphilus Saxus (ca. 1455–1527) was a Modenese poet, author of sonnets and Petrarchesque strambotti. The quotation is from *Elegiarum liber unus*, 2. The quotation is also in Tixier, *Officina*, 2.98 (258).

[18] Perhaps a reference to Athenaeus 13.2. "As for Aristotle of Stageira, did he not beget Nicomachus from the courtesan Herpyllis and live with her until his death? So says Hermippus in the first book of his work *On Aristotle*, adding that she received fitting provision by the terms of the philosopher's will" (6:179).

[19] These first three examples, Aristotle, Nero, and Periander, are from Tixier, *Officina*, 5:64, p. 856. For Nero, see Suetonius, "Nero," 28. Sporos appears earlier in the text.

[20] According to Herodotus, *Histories*, 3:50 (2:63–64). Melissa was Periander's wife.

[21] All of the examples from Semiramis to Xerxes are in Tixier, *Officina*, 5.65 (864–65).

[22] In the edition of *L'hospedale* (Venice: Somascho, 1586) Garzoni has "horse" instead of "bull," indicating a reliance on the original source (Celio, *Lectiones*) rather than

And, according to Volterrano,[23] the shepherd Cratides became enflamed over a she-goat. And, according to Plutarch in his *Parallel Lives*,[24] Aristo of Ephesus fell in love with a female donkey. And, by the same author's testimony, Fulvius, the Roman, fell in love with a mare by whom he sired a daughter named Hippona. Then there's Cyparissus who loved a doe. And Pygmalion and Alciada of Rhodes, both of whom became madly in love with a statue. And then there's Xerxes who became passionately in love with a sycamore tree.[25]

In more modern times, Galeazzo from Mantua—according to the account by Pontano[26]—fell in love with a girl from Pavia. When, as a joke, she told him to go drown himself, he threw himself into the Tesino River.[27] Even more recently, Tirone from Milan fell madly in love with a fish in a fish-pond, which he called The Hunchback. When a company of merry youths had it for dinner, he remained most distressed by his loss for several days. Nor could he be consoled in any way, since it seemed to him that the death of The Hunchback forbode his own iminent demise.

So these are our love-mad fools, commended to the god Cupid,[28] and, in their name, we most affectionately salute him with the following oration:

An Oration to the God Cupid, on Behalf of the Love-Mad

Hail, lovely winged baby! Hail, most gentle son of Venus! Hail, most excellent quivered archer! And once more, Hail! Most crafty warrior in the military actions of love!

Tixier. In addition, Justin (*Ex Trogi Pompeii historiis extensis libri XLIV*) refers to Semiramis but does not mention bestiality, suggesting to Barelli that Garzoni was not always solely dependent on Tixier: Barelli, 110 n. 23.

[23] "Volterrano": Rafaello Maffei, called "Il Volterrano" (1451–1522), scholar whose encyclopedic *Commentariorum rerum urbanarum libri XXXVIII* (Basel: Froben, 1544) was a widely-read compilation in the sixteenth century.

[24] Plutarch, "Greek and Roman Parallel Stories," 29 in Plutarch, *Moralia*, 4:299. Fulvius' story is here too.

[25] "Cyparissus": Ovid, *Metamorphoses*, 10. 108. Cyparissus loved a beautiful stag. He accidentally killed it, and in the course of his morbid grief was turned into a cypress tree. Pygmalion: in Ovid, *Metamorphoses*, 10:81f (243f). Pygmalion fell in love with an ivory statue of a maiden which he himself had carved. The Xerxes story is in Herodotus, *Histories*, 7. 31.

[26] For Pontano, see p. 48, note 25.

[27] In Tixier, *Officina*, 2.98 (274). The "Tesino" is "Ticino" in modern Italian.

[28] Cupid's epithets and attributes can be found in Giraldi, *De deis gentium*, 405–411.

All these fools caught in your net, lured with your bait, imprisoned in your jail, with humble submission pray to you as subjects of your dominion and empire, that you will care about their pain, and have as much pity on their trials and tribulations as would be not only be considered appropriate for a tender, soft-hearted god such as you, but also absolutely fitting and proper. Untie your ropes, take away your hooks, throw away your arrows, lay down your bow, and show yourself to them — disarmed and naked — so that they will not fear those weapons which have already wounded them and have shown them how much damage they can inflict. If you do these things, they promise to make an offering to you, in that famous temple of yours on the island of Cyprus, of a giant chunk of flint without the striking-stone, in order to demonstrate that your flames have been shut up and your fire hidden, which, when it bursts forth, singes everyone's heart.

The Nineteenth Discourse: The Desperate

Certain events sometimes happen to people and have such an effect that they, being deeply affected by the bitterness of these events, precipitously fall into such great despair that, having lost their sense and understanding, they completely give themselves over to sorrow, and consent, with their afflicted and abated spirits, to whatever the severity of their situation—no less stolidly than cruelly—persuades them to believe. From this malignant process, one acquires the name Desperate Madmen among people, because this sort of passion is truly an insanity manifest in those who, unable to tolerate pain, race toward an end that is unworthy of a wise person or one who is able to maintain control over himself.

The first example of this type that occurs to us is Lucius Silanus,[1] son-in-law of the emperor Claudius, who, because he was deprived of his wife Octavia, who had been given to Nero, was suddenly weighted down with such a great sorrow that the very day of their wedding—as envy grew within him, according to Cornelius Tacitus—he killed himself with his own dagger.

The second example is that of Silius Italicus, a famous poet, about whom Angelo Poliziano wrote in his *Nutricia*.[2] When he became afflicted with an incurable disease, he became so despondent that, out of desperation, he committed suicide. These are the verses that were written about him:

Ipse obiit plenusque aevi, natoque superstes,
Aspera congenito fixus vestigia clavo.

---

[1] Lucius Junius Silanus, Roman praetor, was betrothed to Octavia, daughter of the emperor Claudius. But Agrippina, Claudius' wife, wanted her own son, Nero, to marry Octavia. Agrippina arranged to have Silanus dishonored. She then managed to have Nero marry Octavia, and later paved the way for Nero's ascent to the emperorship by murdering Claudius. Knowing that he would soon be killed, Silanus killed himself on the day that Nero and Octavia were married: Tacitus, *Annals*, 12.3–4, and 81, and in Tixier, *Officina*, 2:98 (266–78), as are all of the examples which follow up to "Timanthes."

[2] Poliziano, *Nutricia*, 524–525.

He himself dies full of years, outliving his son,
Cruelly affected by a congenital defect of the feet.[3]

In the *Roman Chronicles* we read of Marcus Portius Latronus[4] who, overwhelmed by a severe case of quartan fever, laid his own hands on himself and ended his life of his own free will.

In Ovid we find the story of Sardanapalus, king of the Assyrians. He was humiliated by a very grievous war, and, when he saw things turning against him, he threw himself in desperation onto a burning pyre and miserably immolated himself in that fire. Ovid wrote:

Inque pyram tecum carissima corpora mittas,
  Quem finem vitae Sardanapalus habet.[5]

And on the pyre were thrown the precious bodies:
This was the way Sardanapalus ended his life.

In modern times, Biondo[6] and Corio[7] both mention Ezzelino, the tyrant of Padua. Having been wounded in battle by the men of Martino Turriano,[8] prince of Milan, he acted like a rabid beast, tearing off his bandages and, desperate man that he was, he vomited up his soul which had been born solely to cause damage and ruin to the human race.

Celio tells this nice story about Timanthes of Cleonae, a professional athlete who—partly because he was old and partly because he had not practiced—was

---

[3] Pliny the Younger, *Epistles,* 3.7, reports that Silius' illness was a disease of his foot (*insanabilis clavus*). See Cherchi, 319, n. 2.

[4] Marcus Portius Latronus, famous Roman rhetorician (55 B.C.-5 A.D.), friend of Seneca the Elder and teacher of Ovid. Tixier, *Officina,* 2:98 (276). The reference is to Eusebius, *Chronici Canones,* 251. Garzoni's text has "Marco Porzio Catone," but Latronus is meant. See Barelli, 114, n. 3.

[5] Ovid, *Ibis,* 311–312. The story is also told in Athenaeus, *Deipnosophistae,* 12.529 (389). Also in Tixier, *Officina,* 2.98 (266).

[6] Biondo: the historian, Flavio Biondo da Forli (1392–1463), author, among other works, of a history of medieval Italy, *Historiarum ab Inclinato Romano imperio decades III* (Basel: Frobeniana, 1531): Fiorato, n. 457.

[7] Corio: Bernardino Corio (1459–1519), courtier at the Sforza court in Milan and historian of the Lombards. His *Patria historia...* (Milan: A. Minutianus, 1503) was one of the first histories written in Italian: Fiorato, n. 457.

[8] Martino Turriano: Martino della Torre II, who was lord of Milan in 1357: Fiorato, n. 458.

unable to draw a bow that a young man could easily handle. Therefore, he got into such despair, because of this, that he killed himself with a knife.[9]

The divine Ariosto located a similar mood in fair Bradamante. But it gets suddenly cast away from her mind by another spirit. The stanza begins:

> Resolved to die 'twas so the damsel cried;
> And starting from her bed, by passion warmed,
> To her left breast her naked sword applied

and all that follows.[10]

In our time, the desperate madness that is described in Cecco of Brisselli is truly ridiculous. He suffered from a noxious mange. As a consequence, in the middle of summer he was mightily annoyed by swarms of flies, as happens in such cases. The annoyance they caused to him was so great, since he was unable to swat them away from his nose or from his forehead or from his hands or from the nape of his neck, which were all encrusted, that one day he threw himself in desperation into a tub of honey, saying, "Now you will remain stuck in here." Then, as he got out of the tub, he saw those nuisances swimming there in the tub, to his great delight. Then look at what happened: attracted by the odor of honey, a troublesome swarm of wasps and bees arrived. He was greatly tormented by their buzzing and stinging and became completely insane due to this second assault. So he dressed himself from head to foot like a soldier at arms, with his visor closed. He sat down in the sun and said, "Now buzz around as much as you want, for despite all of the flies and bees and wasps in the world, I will enjoy my scabies all by myself." But an infinitely large squadron of these creatures were attracted to him because of his odor. At last, unable to watch as he was attacked in this way, he plunged in desperation into a kettle of boiling lye, saying, "So come here, then, and sting me if your love of honey is as great as it seems to be!"[11]

The fools that we have just spoken about are desperate fools. They have for their insignia in our Hospital the image of the goddess Venilia.[12] Therefore, as their champion, we entreat her with the appropriate prayers in their name.

---

[9] Timanthes of Cleonae: famous Greek athlete, many times an Olympic champion; not able to watch himself grow old, he killed himself. The means of suicide vary among the accounts of Celio, *Lectiones,* 626 and Tixier, *Officina,* 2.98 (268).

[10] "All that follows" is that Bradamante, in the midst of trying to stab herself in the side, remembered that she was in full armor: *Orlando Furioso,* 32.44.

[11] The story recalls Aesop, *Fables,* "The Bald Man and the Fly," with its moral, "You will only injure yourself if you take notice of despicable enemies."

[12] Venilia: goddess of the wind and the seas, ally of Neptune, wife of Janus and mother of Turnus, although according to Virgil, *Aeneid,* 10.75, she is the wife of Faunus. This goddess is not mentioned by Giraldi. Cherchi (321, n. 5) speculates she is Garzoni's invention, perhaps evoking the idea of *venia,* or redemption for these suicidal fools.

Supplication to the Goddess Venilia on behalf of the Desperate

O, You who fill the soul with unwavering hope; you who console disconsolate minds with wise thoughts, who restore flagging spirits with pure joy, and who are therefore quickly invoked by all the afflicted—while you look at the other travails and at the wicked suffering of these fools, may your heart, O merciful one, be moved by your great pity, and, making yourself known as the goddess Venilia, Mother of the Desperate,[13] may they be, by your grace, brought back to life as if they had been raised from the dead. For when they see that their lost spirit, their lost blood, and their extinguished color have all been restored, they will be pulled together —with sweet bonds— to hang up in your temple a hangman's noose with a torn reinforcement as a true sign that they have escaped death through your intercession, and have been rescued from a desperate state to having a firm hope for future life.

---

[13] This is also a title of the Virgin Mary: Mother of the Hopeless (Desemparados).

The Twentieth Discourse: The Heteroclites, the Odd, the Lame-Brained, and the Done-For[1]

There are some fantastical temperaments in the world who cannot be persuaded in any way as to what is right nor honest, nor true. They have neither rules, nor order, nor manners to their operations. They have a brain crippled in every region which does not acknowledge their debts, does not agree with what is just, and does not conform with what reason dictates. In everything they do their mind is off the beaten path and far, indeed, from the true way. People with this temperament are always referred to as Heteroclites, Bizarre, Lame-Brained, or Done-for Madmen.

Perseus, defeated by Paulus Aemilius,[2] demonstrated this temperament. While two of his household servants tried to console him in an amicable way following his loss, he worked himself up into such a fit over this that, beast that he was, he commanded, counter to all the reason in the world, that they should be put to death in his presence.[3]

Athenaeus[4] reported that the philosopher Eurylochus, a student of Pyrrho of Elis,[5] was a Done-for Madman because at times he got into such a rage at some trivial incident that he chased one of his cooks all the way to the marketplace, running after him with a spit still holding the steaming-hot roast.

---

[1] Heteroclite: a term borrowed from grammar, where it indicates irregularity.

[2] Paulus Aemilius, called "The Macedonian" (ca. 230–160 B.C.), proconsul and Roman general who defeated Perseus, king of Macedonia, at Pydna in 168 B.C. On his victorious return to Rome, he was granted a three-day triumph. According to Plutarch (*Lives,* 6:41) Perseus was enraged by the censure and unreasonably bold speeches of two of his treasurers and therefore killed them by his own hand: Tixier, *Officina,* 2.21 (116).

[3] All of the episodes in this section are found in Tixier, *Officina,* 5.25, "Of Rage and Hatred" (748–49).

[4] The anecdote is not in *The Deipnosophists.* See Diogenes Laertius, *Life of Pyrrho,* 7.

[5] Pyrrho of Elis is the Greek philosopher (365–275 B.C.), founder of the school of Skeptics. Discussed by Diogenes Laërtius, *Vitae philosophorum,* 9.68.

Many authors have written about this great affair regarding the emperor Commodus.[6] He once discovered that the bath water that he was about to use was tepid, and, in a mighty rage, he threw the servant who was tending the fire into a raging furnace so that while he was taking his tepid bath, the fire-tender would feel just the opposite, the heat which his spiteful insanity had given to him.

Sansovino[7] writes about Mehmed the Ottoman who, while strolling in his garden, happened to notice that two of his beautiful watermelons had been picked off their plants. He accused two pretty boys with most elegant figures (whom he had also abused as lovers) and, even though they denied having done it, he most cruelly murdered them on the spot.

Philagros the sophist, who was a student of Lollianus,[8] also had a brain that was so odd and heteroclite that if his students — solely out of necessity — ever fell asleep in class, he would not excuse their need of it, but would go over and punch them in the face and kick them in the stomach without the least compassion for the necessities of nature.

It is clear from what Biondo[9] has written, that Vedius Pollio[10] was a Done-for Madman in everything that he did. If one of his servants happened to break even one of his cheapest glasses, he would immediately, as if in an insane fury, command that they be killed and fed to the lampreys which he kept in one of his fish ponds, remarkable for their enormous size.

Chaerephon of Athens, a little-known philosopher, was so much a madman of this type that, when talking about a Done-for Madman, Paolo Manuzio gave birth to this proverb:

---

[6] Commodus: also mentioned in Discourses XIIII (p. 112, note 17) and XVIII (p. 129, note 6). The source is *Scriptores Historiae Augustae*, "Commodus," 1.9, trans. Magie, 1:267.

[7] Sansovino: Francesco Sansovino (1521–1586), Venetian politician, writer, and historiographer, and author, among other works, of a history of the Turks, *Historia universale dell'origine del regno et imperio de' Turchi* (Venice: F. Rampazzetto, 1564). Fiorato (n. 473) identifies Mehmed the Ottoman as Mehmed II.

[8] Lollianus of Ephesus, Greek sophist at the time of Hadrian (second century A.D.). Garzoni's two principal sources, Tixier, *Officina*, 5.25 (748) and Celio, *Lectiones*, 804 differ in their telling of this story. For Philagros, see Tixier, *Officina*, 5.25 (747). Philostratus, who recorded the anecdote in *Lives of the Sophists* (207–15), describes him as "the most excitable and hot-tempered of the sophists."

[9] Biondo: see 138 n. 6 above.

[10] Vedius Pollio (d. 15 B.C.) was a friend of Augustus. The anecdote (Seneca, *De Ira*, 3.40; Dio Cassius, *Roman History*, 54.23) refers to an incident which occurred when Augustus was dining with Pollio. The slave appealed to the emperor, but Pollio was not swayed. Augustus then ordered all of Pollio's crystal to be broken and his fish pond to be filled in.

In Palladis vestigiis nihil Cherofontis gubernabis.

Following Pallas, one can never control Chaerephon.[11]

The singular example of the oddness of Bernabò Visconti can be found in Corio.[12] He had a poor baker slain solely because at night, when he passed by the castle where Visconti lived to deliver his bread, the baker, delivering his bread, would sometimes awaken him when he cried out that he had bread.

That other story about him is well-known to everyone. He forced two of the Holy Father's representatives to eat the letters that they had brought for him, solely out of spite for the pontiff with whom he was having public hostilities regarding matters of state.

Nor does what Visconti did to that priest (who, by the way, deserved severe punishment for his avarice) lack the flavor of leeks:[13] Because he was unwilling to bury a poor woman's husband for free, Visconti made the priest lie down in the grave with the dead man as payment for the iniquity he had committed in public.

So these are the Done-For or Odd, Heteroclite Madmen that we have described. Above their cell in our Hospital, they keep the image of lame Vulcan,[14] crippled in his legs just as they are crippled in their brains. Therefore we properly commend them to a god with whom they have so much in common, with the following oration:

---

[11] In other words, "If you follow the path of Pallas Athena, goddess of Intelligence and Wisdom, you will never be able to control the madness of Chaerephon." This is probably the parasite described by Athenaeus, *Deipnosophists*, 5.244–45 (3:93 ff).

[12] The anecdotes of Bernabò Visconti (1323–1385) are not to be found in Corio, but his cruelty is discussed in the *Storia di Milano*, part 3, p. 588 ff. of the Venetian edition of 1564. The episodes reported by Garzoni are derived from short stories, beginning with *Trecento novelle*, 59, by Sacchetti, who tells the story of the priest. See V. Vitali, "Bernabò Visconti nella novella e nella cronaca contemporanea," *Archivio Storico Lombardo*, 15 (1901): 261–85. One finds Garzoni's specific sources in this tradition. For example, the episode of the furnace can be found in G. Bugati, *Historia universale*, Book 7, p. 272 of the Venetian edition of 1571. The story of Innocent's legates can be found in L. Domenichi, *Historia varia* (Venezia: Giolito, 1564), 427–28. Domenichi reports that Visconti met the two legates on the bridge at Lambro and said, "Do you want to be thrown into the river, or do you want to eat the letters?" They ate them. The story of the priest is in Domenichi, *Historia*, 317. See Cherchi, 323, n. 5 and Fiorato, n. 479.

[13] I.e., this one is also comical. See Fiorato, 302, note 483.

[14] Vulcan, god of fire and furnaces, often represented as lame, as Garzoni explains in the Oration to him. His attributes are to be found in Giraldi, *De deis gentium*, 13 (413–17).

An Oration to the God Vulcan on Behalf of Odd Heteroclites, the Lame-Brained, and the Done-for

We pray to you, O Great Celestial Smith, Minister of Fire for Mt. Aetna, called Mulciber because you make iron malleable; Vulcan, because you cause your flames to fly speedily aloft; Cyllopodius, because when you fell from the heavens in disgrace, you unfortunately came up lame; Lemnius, because when your mother threw you down from heaven, you landed in Lemnos where you were nourished by Eurynome and Thetis[15] — or perhaps by apes. So, just as you usually do — with the same pity that was shown you in your disaster at that time — assist, with pity, these brothers of yours, lame not in their legs but, as you can see, lame in their brains. And just as you temper Jupiter's thunderbolts; and just as you put together the nets that caught Venus and Mars; and just as you made Hermione's necklace; and just as you made Ariadne's crown; and just as you made the Sun's chariot; and just as you, with your own hands, forged the arms of Achilles and Aeneas in the furnaces of the Cyclopes; just as you made Mambrino's helmet, and Orlando's Durindana, and Rinaldo's Fusberta, the magical arms of Mandricardo, and Argalia's armor;[16] in the same way temper the brains of these madmen so that, in triumph, they can hang inside your shop a gigantic Lombard stew,[17] which will serve as a sign of these men's tidy brains which, through you, have been reduced to that true-tempered state which they need.

---

[15] This story of being nourished by Eurynome and Thetis is not in Giraldi. Garzoni has "Eurymone." Cherchi guesses that "Hermione" rather than "Eurymone" is meant, a reference to the famous necklace that Vulcan made for her, although Hermione's necklace is referred to just a few lines later: Cherchi, 324, n. 7. Eurynome and Thetis were two marine divinities who rescued Vulcan after he was cast off by his mother, Hera, so Eurynome is most likely meant.

[16] Mambrino's helmet: the golden helmet of the Saracen warrior; the object of one of Don Quixote's quests. In chapter 21, Quixote mistakes a barber's shaving basin for the helmet. Mambrino's helmet and all the other items appear in Ariosto's *Orlando Furioso*. Orlando's Durindana is his mythic sword reputedly having belonged first to Hector. Rinaldo's Fusberta is his sword. Mandricardo wears the helmet and armor of Hector. Argalia's remarkable helmet was lost in a stream.

[17] Cervelletto, a term applied to several different gastronomic dishes as, for example, in Messisburgo, *Libro di cucina* (Venice: Padoano, 1557). The word plays on "*cervellino*," or "scatter-brain": Cherchi, 324, n. 10.

The Twenty-First Discourse: The Buffoons

Fables, babble, tales that, I must say, are expressed not cleverly but comically, together with similar actions, gestures, and activities constitute that sort of madman that we term the Buffoon. Their intent is nothing more than to provide amusement to the world, since they have a certain mental disposition beyond joviality which oppresses them in such a way that they say and do a thousand sillinesses every day before the crowd.

Take Clisophus, for example, a parasite of Philip, king of Macedon,[1] about whom Lynceus of Samos[2] writes in his *Commentaries*. Observing that his master had broken his leg in an accident, he started to limp just like him and would squinch up his eyes, his mouth, and his teeth when he ate tart things, thus, like a monkey, diligently aping his master.

Furthermore, according to Hegesander,[3] one can find this written about Charisophus, jester to the tyrant Dionysius:[4] whenever he saw his master with certain barons or noblemen laughing among themselves, he would also laugh with great gusto, so that one day, Dionysius, noticing his clown, asked him why he was laughing. To which the clown replied, "I laugh for this reason: because I imagine that the things that you talk about together deserve to be laughed at, seeing as how you laugh the way you do."

---

[1] Philip of Macedon (382–336 B.C.), father of Alexander. Clisophus (or Cleisophus) also "covered one of his eyes with a bandage out of compliment to Philip who had lost an eye at the siege of Methone": Aelian, *Characteristics of Animals*, 9.7 (2.229).

[2] Lynceus of Samos, Greek author of comedies, fourth-third centuries B.C. These two anecdotes are in Tixier, *Officina*, 5.40.

[3] Hegesander of Delphi (second century B.C.), author of a collection of anecdotes. Hegesander said this "in honor" of philosophers: "Sons-of-eyebrow-raisers, noses-fixed-in-beards, beards-bag-fashion-trimmed, and casserole-pilferers too, cloaks-over-shoulders-slinging, barefoot-shambling-with-eyes-cast-down, night-birds-secretly-feeding, night-sinners-in-deceit, puny-lad-deceivers, and silly-brothers-of-sought-syllables, wise-in-their-vain-conceits, degenerate-sons-of-seekers-after-good." Quoted in Athenaeus, *Deipnosophists*, 4.162 (2: 237).

[4] Dionysius, tyrant of Syracuse (405–367 B.C.) The story is found in Celio, *Lectiones*, 795 and 866, but is also in Tixier, *Officina*, 5.40 (781).

But above all, Marcus Varro[5] and Galba[6] mention a certain vile clown from Tarentum called Rhynthon,[7] who was like Cesco[8] in our own time, because for everything that he did, no matter how grave or serious, he always had a ready jest which, for him, might have been like his mother or sister.

Similarly, Sosicrates,[9] in the first book of his *On Things Cretan*, attributes the characteristic of buffoonery to the Phaestians,[10] because from the time they were small children, they carefully studied many clever sayings in order to sharpen their wits, which were greatly improved by this practice.

In ancient times, Mandrogenes[11] and Straton of Athens were famous clowns, as Hippolochus of Macedon testifies in the letter which he wrote to Lynceus.[12] So too were Callimedon the Crayfish, Deinias, and Menaechmus. Telephanes,[13] in his book *On the City*, tells that Philip of Macedon owned these clowns and asked them for their counsel. Among still others were Cassiodorus and Pantaleon, glorified by Dionysius of Sinope,[14] the comic poet, and by the poet Theognetus,[15] in his *"He Liked His Master,"* respectively.[16]

These are the ones who sweep the floors of the courts of princes and gentlemen—those who generally enjoy this sort of fool. According to Athenaeus, in the fourteenth book of his *The Deipnosophists*,[17] Philip, king of Macedon, would sometimes give a gold talent to those jesters we have named above as a reward for their witty sayings.

---

[5] Marcus Terentius Varro (116–27 B.C.), prolific man of letters and politician whose encyclopedic works are a major source of information on writers of and before his time.

[6] Servius Sulpicius Galba, famous orator of the Republic: Fiorato, n. 498.

[7] Rhynthon: author of farces, now lost: Tixier, *Officina*, 5.40 (782).

[8] Cesco: a clown contemporary of Garzoni.

[9] Sosicrates of Rhodes, historiographer, author of a book on Crete and of a history of ancient philosophy. The anecdote is in Athenaeus, *Deipnosophists*, 6.261 (3:177).

[10] Phaestians: inhabitants of Phaestos, town in Crete.

[11] Garzoni has "Mandiogene."

[12] As reported in Athenaeus, *Deipnosophists*, 14.614 (6:309).

[13] Telephanes of Samos, celebrated flautist and choir director. Friend of Philip of Macedon. He was praised by Demosthenes for his loyalty. The material in this paragraph, including the reference to Telephanes' book *On the City of Athens*, is found in Athenaeus, *Deipnosophists*, 14.614 (6:311), although Athenaeus has "Cephissodorus," not "Cassiodorus."

[14] Dionisius of Sinope, Greek poet (middle of the fifth century B.C.).

[15] Theognetus or Theognis: Greek gnomic poet from Megara (fifth century B.C.). This paragraph is derived from Athenaeus, *Deipnosophists*, 14 (6:317).

[16] The paragraph comes from Athenaeus, *Deipnosophists*, 14. 615–616 (6:317).

[17] Athenaeus, *Deipnosophists*, 14.615–616.

According to Phylarchus,[18] in the sixth book of his *Histories*,[19] Demetrius Poliorcetes was such a great friend of clowns that he could never send them away. Similarly, Herodotus wrote that Amasis, king of Egypt, loved the company of clowns more than that of the wise and virtuous.[20] But this is an amazing thing: Nicostratus,[21] in the twenty-seventh book of his *Histories*, attributes this same genius to the Roman, Sulla, who was otherwise so serious and so grave in his affairs.

In our time, both Gonella[22] and Carafulla were the greatest of clowns. Even more recently, the Paduan Boccafresca[23]—who, I believe, has no peer, let alone was surpassed for buffoonery—was so much more a clown by never laughing even though he made everyone else laugh. He was not unlike the people of Tiryns celebrated by Theophrastus, who, being born clowns, once called on the Oracle of Delphi to learn if it were possible to become free of this sort of madness. The Oracle responded that it would be if they were able to sacrifice a bull to Neptune, god of the sea, without laughing. But they couldn't do it, so they stayed in the same state of buffoonery as they had before.[24]

Clowns are at least good for this: that they make people happy and cast out melancholy from their breasts. Nor do they break bread deceitfully the way flatterers do, from whom nothing is gained but both injury and disgrace.

These madmen have erected an image of the god Fabulanus, their friend, above their cell in our Hospital. So it should not be surprising if we duly and properly commend them to him, who is the protector of these fabulous chatterers, with the following oration:

---

[18] Phylarchus: little-known Greek historian. He is the author of a history covering the period between Philip of Macedon and Ptolemy Philopator: Tixier, *Officina*, 5.24, "On Arrogance, Pride, and Ambition" (743). This and the following anecdotes regarding clowns are found in Athenaeus, *Deipnosophists*, 6.261 (3:177).

[19] Actually, the tenth book, not the sixth.

[20] Herodotus, *Histories*, 2. 173–175. Also reported in Athenaeus, *Deipnosophists*, 6.261 (3:171).

[21] According to Athenaeus, *Deipnosophists*, 6.261 (3:175), the citation should be to "the one hundred and seventh book of his histories."

[22] Gonella: famous Florentine clown of the fourteenth century, in the service of Obizzo II d'Este. His exploits were chronicled by many authors, including F. Sacchetti and M. Bandello. See Fiorato, n. 509.

[23] We have no information on Carafulla and Boccafresca.

[24] Athenaeus, *Deipnosophists*, 6.261 (3:177) explains: "They forbade their children from attending the sacrifice, but one boy learned what was going on, and mingling with the crowd, he cried out, 'What's the matter with you? Are you afraid I shall upset your victim?' At this, they burst into laughter."

An Oration to the god Fabulanus[25] on behalf of Buffoons

These men, O God Fabulanus, are true buffoons, friends and partisans for life of your name. For they have nothing in their ears, nor have anything on their tongues but fables and tall tales which are born from you, and, inserted into them, take such strong roots that they show themselves to be the children and true descendants of the great god Fabulanus. Because of this, it is right that your deity, glorified by the kings of this world, should take custody of your dear friends and hold them in such great esteem because they know that, without you, they would be unable to say anything at all that was witty or charming. So assure them of their requisite protection and do it in such a way that they can make an offering to you at the altar which you have among the people of Tiryns, a Piovano Arlotto,[26] printed on parchment, in big letters, so that the donation or present which they give to you aptly matches their courteous and generous benefactor.

---

[25] Fabulanus: according to Fiorato (n. 513), a reference to the Roman god Fabulinus, who was invoked to bring speech to babies. Cherchi finds little similarity between Garzoni's creation and this god, however (327, n. 11).

[26] See page 94, note 7 above.

The Twenty-Second Discourse: The Merry, Sweet, Facetious, and Loving

One can distinguish this type of madman from mere Buffoons by this: Comical Madmen are always ready—without rules, without moderation, and without discretion—to speak and perform all sorts of licentious buffoonery; but the Facetious ones not only are not so extreme in their speech and actions, they also observe a modicum of decorum and style in everything they do. The merriment of their choruses is much more tempered than that of the Comical ones which is absolutely dissolute. They are generally full of jolly quips, graceful tales, enjoyable sayings, nonsense proverbs, and polished witticisms, and they seem, in their outward appearance, to show to everyone a cozy nature—friendly, sweet, affable—and with a delightful wit.

Marcus Tullius, in a letter to his brother Quintus, wrote that Sextus Naevius[1] was one of these, and in the second section of his *On Laws*,[2] included the ancient poet Aristophanes among those having a facetious mind. Similarly, Horace, in the first of his *Sermons*, attributed facetiousness to the poet Lucilius:

Fuerit Lucilius inquam
Comis, et urbanus, fuerit limatior idem.

We must admit that Lucilius was gentle and urbane
And was also most elegant.[3]

---

[1] Cherchi (328, n. 2) indicates that Garzoni has confused this man with Gnaeus Naevius, ancient author of theatrical works, about which Cicero wrote in *Brutus*, 19.76, as well as Gellius, *Attic Nights*, 1.34, where he alludes specifically to his "facetious" spirit. Naevius wrote this for his own epitaph: "If that immortals might for mortals weep / Then would divine Muses weep for Naevius / For after he to Orcus' own treasure consigned / The Romans straight forgot to speak the Latin tongue": Gellius, *Attic Nights*, 1.24 (trans. Rolfe, 1:109). Barelli suggests that Sesto Nevio refers to a flute or trumpet to which Cicero (*Pro Publio Quintio* 3.11) attributed a facetious spirit: Barelli, 125, n. 1.

[2] *De legibus*, 2.15.17.

[3] Horace, *Satires*, 1.10.64–65.

In our day, Piovano Arlotto[4] was reputed to be a wonderfully merry fellow, whose published works and sayings demonstrate to what extent people valued his mind for this sort of foolery. These days, there is no lack of this sort of fool in Rome and at the major courts of nobles, because more courtiers study this sort of thing than any other. It is a most effective means of obtaining the favor of princes and ladies, who are frequently more captivated by some merry nonsense tale than by the long service given by these impertinent souls who, after carefully examining their errors, frequently sing, "O errant footsteps, O soft, frail thoughts."[5]

An example demonstrating this observation is Mr. Bernardino da Benevento who, while serving at the court of a great Italian prince, one day obtained the favor of a beautiful lady solely because of this finely-honed quip: she had said that it felt very hot in her rooms, and he replied, with surprise, "How is that possible, My Lady, since nothing comes from Benevento that is not wonderfully cool!"[6]

Another courtier called Mister Andrea Pomerano, while serving at the court of Francis the First, king of France, obtained for himself the instant favor of his lord with this improvised invention: The court was uncertain about where Charles the Fifth would attack the kingdom of France—some saying it would be from Marseilles, some from Navarre, and still others from Provence, some from one place, some from another. The man said, in the presence of many people, and so that the king could hear, that it was necessary to fortify Languedoc more than any other place, because it was certain that the predatory eagle would attack the "land where oc is spoken" before any other.[7]

About Master Nicoletto of Orvieto[8] this story is told: One day, while serving at the court of Pope Leo, a most courteous pontiff, he obtained the eternal favor of His Holiness with just four words. One day, while they were discussing a vacant benefice which was being sought by someone of the house of Vitelli, with whom Nicoletto had been able to confer, he said wittily, "Holy Father, it is right that it be conferred on Vitello, because it has no relation more near and dear to it."[9]

Merry fools of this type have hanging over their cell in our Hospital a picture of the god Bacchus, special patron of fools like this. Therefore we merrily salute him as their greatest friend with the following jolly oration:

---

[4] See p. 94, note 7.

[5] Roughly based on Petrarch, *Canzoniere*, 161, line 1: "O useless steps, O thoughts charming and quick" *(O passi sparsi, o pensier vaghi et pronti)*.

[6] A play on "Benevento," meaning "pleasant breezes."

[7] Charles V, represented by the predatory eagle, would be most likely to attack the land of the oc, or goose. "Oca" or "goose" is another name for a simpleton or fool.

[8] Nicoletto of Orvieto: he is included in Castiglione's *Book of the Courtier*, 2.66.

[9] The punning plays on *vacante* or "vacant" and *vacca* or "cow" and also *Vitelli*, the family name, and *vitello*, or "calf." It is right that the vacancy be conferred on the Vitelli family, because there is no relationship more near and dear than that between a cow and its calf.

An Oration to the God Bacchus on Behalf of the Merry, Sweet, Facetious, and Loving

Good Day and Good Year, O Father Liber![10] All the joy of the world be with you, my dear god. May a toast be raised to you with muscatel or vernaccia, O sweet Lyaeus! Serve and protect this joyful collegium, consecrated to you. See how they all wait to receive that joy from you which the Bacchic Ladies[11] have had from you, driven madly in love when they followed you so happily to that favorable action in India. As you returned victorious, you were the first one in the naval triumph—which you discovered—to wear the royal diadem while sitting atop an Indian elephant.[12] So if you continue to be their friend, just as you always have been, according to your nature which inclines you toward their kind, they will not content themselves with calling you only Bimater, because you have had—truly miraculously—two mothers in this world, Semele and Jupiter; or of calling you Satumiterus because you were first in her belly and then in his thigh;[13] or of naming you Nyseus of Nysa's Cave; Aonius of Aonia; Thyoneus from Thyon; Nyctelius because you were worshipped and celebrated at night; Mitrophoros, for carrying the mitre on your head; Oreos, from the hill where they make sacrifices to you; Bassaris, from the robe that you wear all the way down to your heels; Dithyrambus, Lenaeus and Brisaeus, Osiris and Bromius,[14] but they would like to give you the name Eutrapelus—in Greek—because you are the favorite of merry, sweet, and facetious fools. In addition to the thyrsis[15] which you carry in your hand, they want to add a jug of romania wine with which you can reason with them when—jolly fellows that they are—they seek you out.

---

[10] All of the epithets for Bacchus—except Satumiterus—are taken from Giraldi, *De deis gentium* 8 (267–90).

[11] The Bacchantes, inebriated by wine's delirium.

[12] A reference to Bacchus' (Dionysus') expedition to India, where he taught the Indians how to grow wine. His trip is variously reported to have lasted from three to 52 years. Diodorus describes three gods with this name, one of whom was born in India: *Diodorus*, trans. Oldfather, 4.3 (2:347).

[13] Bacchus was first carried by his mother, Semele, but when she was burned up by his father, Jupiter, he was removed from his mother's womb and stitched into the thigh of Jupiter, who carried him to term. Giraldi has the story, but not the epithet here used by Garzoni.

[14] Garzoni's text has "Bormius."

[15] "Thyrsis," the long staff entwined with vines that is Bacchus' symbol and the symbol of life and fecundity.

The Twenty-Third Discourse: The Capricious and Frenzied

Capriciousness is a sort of condition caused by fantastical humors which those who are commonly termed Capricious and Frenzied Fools have in their heads. It seems that all of this sort of matter is fomented by rage and human inconstancy. It consists of nothing other than changing their minds and actions, that finally resolve into something eccentric and capricious that is in keeping with someone with these passions. All those who are quick to anger and easy to calm down are of this nature. So the poet Horace showed himself to be a Capricious Fool when he said:

Irasci facilem, tantum ut placabilis essem[1]

Easy to anger, so that I can be calmed down.

And the poet Ausonius, based on his own testimony, was also a Capricious Fool, proffering these verses about himself:

Irasci promptus properavi condere motum
  Atque mihi poenas pro levitate dedi.[2]

Being quick of temper, I made haste to quash this impulse
And punished myself for this weakness of mine.

Cotys, king of Thrace[3] (if Celio does not lie), knowing his own capricious and frenzied nature and how precipitous and impetuous he could be, was once given some beautiful, well-crafted vases which were very dear to him. Thinking about how fragile they were, after careful consideration he smashed all of them. For if

---

[1] Horace, *Epistles*, 1.20.25. See also Tixier, *Officina*, 5.25, where one can also find the references to Ausonius and Cotys. The original version has "Irasci celerem tamen ut placabilis essem," "Quick to anger, nevertheless, easily calmed down."

[2] Ausonius, "An Elegy upon My Father," lines 35–36, in *Ausonius*, trans. Evelyn White, 1:45; modified.

[3] One of a line of kings of Thrace with this name; probably the Cotys who ruled B.C. 382–358, particularly infamous for his brutality: Tixier, *Officina* 5.25 (212).

they had been smashed by one of his servants or assistants it would have been impossible for him, full of rage, not to extract bitter revenge from them.

The divine Ariosto has portrayed the great Rodomonte in this way, because, being capricious and frenzied, he spoke evil of the entire female sex when the lovely Doralice pronounced sentence against him. Yet just at the sight of Isabella, it seems that he recanted, not knowing any other good than her beauty and grace.[4]

In our time, Claudio of Salò[5] proved to be very capricious. Owner of a country house inherited from his father, he decided one day to turn the whole thing into a dovecote. Then, a few days later, he got the feeling that it should be a fortress with ramparts all around and a moat and keeps. As soon as it was finished, his mood changed, and he tore it down to its foundations, then planted a lovely little grove of oranges in its place. But one day, when they had grown into sizable trees, he uprooted them all, on a whim, saying that it would be better if it were a field of cabbages. In this way, his house finally turned into a patch of cabbage-heads.[6]

The capricious temperament of Zanfardino, our contemporary, is also worth noting. Selected for a high office at a time when cuckoos were prized as if they were parrots[7] (even now one sees some expert quips escape from the mouths of their successors),[8] as he took up his position, he began to sell herds of cattle in order to buy geese and he wrecked the gardens to make pens for the geese, rationalizing his capriciousness by saying that geese produce feathers from which one can make pillows and mattresses which he needed more than he needed meat, fruit, and cheese.

Another man, a fellow called Scarinzo whose temperament was no less incredible than the others', tore down a grape arbor with beautiful productive fruit solely to gain an empty, narrow perspective for his idiocy. And when he didn't have anything else to do, he knocked down an outhouse and made a loo out of it; or destroyed a garden in order to make a courtyard; or ruined a portico so he could make a rabbit hutch.

But celebrated above all the other capricious ones is that man from Piacenza who threw gold coins into the sea in order to enjoy the infantile pleasure of watching them flicker like fish. He was so entranced by his pleasure that he wasn't aware of his loss, because of the capricious pride he felt in his brain.

Capricious above all other capricious ones was that man from Cremona who, one day, dressed in the *toga praetexta* or ceremonial robe of a doctor, heard a drummer boy playing the drum very badly, so he came down and took the drum in his hands and loudly banged on it and, scantily clothed, he went into the

---

[4] Ariosto, *Orlando Furioso*, 27.94 ff.

[5] Salò, on the west shore of Lake Garda.

[6] A play on "cabbages" as "fools."

[7] From a proverb: "When cuckoos were valued as much as parrots," meaning, an imaginary time: Fiorato, n. 554. Garzoni also plays on "cuckoo" as meaning "fool."

[8] Meaning that there are still cuckoos around in Garzoni's time.

square beating it and attracting swarms of little boys and everybody's attention, causing so much laughter at his foolishness that they could have all died.

An even more noteworthy deed was that by a man nicknamed The Muscovite.[9] He was giving a funeral oration for a doctor in the town of Bracciano.[10] He leaped to the pulpit full of grandeur and dressed in full armor, rested his spear and, in the loftiest of tones, said, "If anyone would be so impudent as to say that this doctor died a good death and that Fate cut short the thread of his life with good cause, I will challenge him to combat with me, and with this lance in my hand, I will fight to the death, right at this pulpit."

I offer this next example solely for the entertainment of the crowd. There was once a certain Nicolò of Monte Frustone[11] who was so whimsical that one day, when he happened to be on the banks of the Po while the miller was away, he unfastened one of those mills which stand tied up in the water. The mill floated downstream with the current, and he followed it in a little boat from Stellata to Francolino[12] where he drove it aground, almost completely smashed and destroyed. Then he ordered a huge hole to be dug so that it could be buried, and then paid twelve old women to mourn for it as if they were at a funeral, saying these words:

> Oh, poor mill
> Laid to rest at Francolino,
> What did you do to Nicolò
> To make him let you loose?
> We will always mourn for you,
> Since we will have no flour.
> Oh woe, oh woe, oh woe,
> Bread is worth more than brains!

So these are all our capricious fools who have in front of their cell in our Hospital a Tisiphone[13] for their sign because she is the goddess of their temperament. Therefore we pray to ask for her help for them with the following oration:

---

[9] "Muscovite": a play on *mosco*, or "fly."

[10] Bracciano: small town in Latium, north of Rome, near the lake of the same name.

[11] Monte Frustone. The town cannot be located. Perhaps a creation of Garzoni's, from *frusto*, meaning shabby and threadbare.

[12] Stellata, Francolino: two small towns on the Po near Ferrara.

[13] Tisiphone: one of the three Erinyes or Furies, violent goddesses of hatred and avengers of murder: Giraldi, *De deis gentium*, 209–17.

A Petition to Tisiphone on Behalf of the Capricious and Frenzied

O, You, cruel in heaven, furious on earth, Eumenid in hell, great daughter of Night and of Acheron, take away from them some of your whimsical fury, because unfortunately they are sometimes capricious and furious. If you want them to offer you in secret a pair of pigeons at your temple in Athens—as agreeable as they are—who, because of this, have been dedicated to you a thousand times before: this will show the world that these capricious bears, enticed by your beneficence as if by a tidbit of honey, can sometimes become like little lambs.

The Twenty-Fourth Discourse:
The Violent and Beastly: In Need of Ropes and Chains

Among the race of fools, none are more unbearable than those that we call Violent or Beastly, because the properties of their brains are so wild and reckless that it is necessary to run from them just as you would from the frenzy of unrestrained, cursed beasts. Nor are they only insane towards others on whom they inflict damage with all the beastliness that dominates them; they also turn this frenzy against themselves, as the frenzy directs their brains towards every sort of evil that can be imagined.

Ancient Hercules is depicted with this sort of frenzy. After he put on the tunic of the centaur Nessus, impatient with sorrow, he threw himself into the flames of Mount Oeta. So Claudian sang:

Iuga deseris Oetes,
Herculeo damnata rogo.

Thou quittest the heights of Oeta,
Condemned as Hercules' funeral pyre.[1]

In the thirteenth book of the *Metamorphoses*, Ovid describes Ajax, son of Telamon, as being ravished by that same frenzy because the Greeks decreed that Achilles' arms should be given to Ulysses rather than to him.[2]

Similarly, Ariosto uniquely describes Orlando's frenzied insanity in two particular verses. The first one says:

Drawing his sword, he slashed the offending rock,
And heavenwards the splintered fragments flew.[3]

And in the other, he says:

---

[1] Claudian, *Panegyric on the Third Consulship of the Emperor Honorius*, 1.114–115 (trans. Platnauer, 1:279), revised. Also in Tixier, *Officina*, 2.98.

[2] Ovid, *Metamorphoses*, 13.380–398. Also in Tixier, *Officina*, 2.60. Ajax killed himself when Achilles' arms were given to Ulysses: the subject of the tragedy *Ajax* by Sophocles.

[3] Ariosto, *Orlando Furioso*, trans. Rose, 23.130.1–2.

> With tree-trunks, branches, stones, and clods of earth
> He sullies the fair waters of the stream,
> Choking and clouding them for all he's worth,
> From top to bottom, murky now and dim.[4]

And this is why elsewhere he describes how, when Astolfo wanted to heal him, he had to tie him up with many ropes, like a chained-up crazy, which is what he had become.[5]

Athamas, son of Aeolus, was described by Ovid as very beastly and frenzied to the point that, in his violent temper, he murdered his own son who was called Learchus. In the sixth book of his *Fasti*, Ovid writes:

> *Hinc agitur furiis Athamas sub imagine falsa*
> *tuque cadis patria parve Learche manu.*[6]

> So Athamas is haunted by false appearances and by the Furies;
> And you, little Learchus, die by the hand of your father.

Herodotus writes this about Cambyses:[7] having violated the Egyptian god Apis, he was transformed into such a frenzy that first, stirred up by the Furies, he murdered almost his entire family and then, turning his wrath on himself, he insanely killed himself.

Propertius,[8] in his third book, places Alcmaeon, son of Amphiaraus and Eriphyle, among the Furious Fools. Having murdered his mother, he was led and driven by her fixed image into this sort of madness. So he writes of him,

> *Aut Alcmeoniae furiae, aut jejunia Phinei*

> Either Alcmaeon by the furies, or Phineas by hunger.

---

[4] Ariosto, *Orlando Furioso*, trans. Rose, 23.104.3–8.

[5] Ariosto, *Orlando Furioso*, trans. Rose, 39.54–55.

[6] Ovid, *Fasti*, 6.6.489–90. Tixier, *Officina* 2.60, "On the Furious and Maniacal" (213). See also Garzoni, *Teatro*, Disc. 52, n. 2.

[7] Cambyses II, king of Persia (ca. 528–521 B.C.). Cruel ruler, considered a fool for his military defeats in Africa. After killing the sacred bull of Apis, he killed his mother, tried to marry his sister, did marry another sister, and killed the first one. He assassinated his son and committed suicide out of despair (although according to other sources, he died accidentally): Herodotus, *Histories*, 3.27–38, 61–66; Tixier, *Officina*, 2.60 (212). Seneca, *Epistles*, 86.1, thought that Cambyses was mad, but made "successful use of his madness" by showing moderation and a sense of duty.

[8] Propertius, *Elegies*, 3.5.41; Tixier, *Officina*, 2.60 (214). Propertius muses on his old age, when he will study the great questions about nature, including whether Alcmaeon was plagued by furies and Phineas by hunger.

In his first book, Lucan[9] numbers a certain Pentheus among this type of madman because, having been disrespectful to the god Bacchus, he was punished by him by making Pentheus furious and crazy like an animal:

Nec magis attonitos animi sensere tumultus
cum fureret Pentheus, aut cum descisset Agave.

Nor did Pentheus in his madness, or Agave, when she returned to her senses,
Feel more horror and disturbance of mind.

Celio wrote that Orestes, son of Agamemnon and Clytemnestra, after he had murdered his mother, became mad and tore off all of his clothes and bit off one of his own fingers.[10] Paolo Manuzio devised this proverb: "To weave Orestes' tunic,"[11] which is said about someone who gives a man a present that he will eventually misuse.

In our time, a certain soldier of Brisighella[12] was a great Furious Fool. He fell furiously in love with a girl from Faventa and then ate a gauntlet and an armor breastplate at one sitting. Beastly passions had risen so high into the vault of his brain that he was no longer able to tell the difference between his breastplate and his bread.

Cambles, king of Lydia, was similar to him, if Celio is right. One night, while possessed by a furor of gluttony, he ate his wife who was lying next to him. In the morning, finding one of her hands in his mouth, he became truly insane, like a chained beast.[13]

The example of Santin of Villafranca[14] is not without style. He became enraged when one of his cows and one of his bulls died, so he went to his neighbor's stable where there were a donkey, a sow, and several piglets. Possessed by this fury, he killed them all and ate half of the donkey without taking a single drink.

Another one, called Marchione of Buffalora near Milan, who was an altar boy for a certain priest from Varese, fell into this beastly temperament because one of his candles had been stolen by a rogue. So he ran to the belltower and ate almost an entire bell-clapper, providing the community with no less entertainment than damage when they learned about it.

---

[9] Lucan, *Pharsalia.*, 7.780–781, Tixier; *Officina*, 2.60 (212–13).

[10] Garzoni cites Celio, but the example is in Tixier, *Officina*, 2.60 (212).

[11] Manuzio, *Adagia* (1024) and Erasmus, *Adagia*, 4.1.48.

[12] Brisighella, a small town on the border between Emilia Romagna and Tuscany, about 20 miles south of Bagnacavallo, Garzoni's home town.

[13] Celio, *Lectiones*, 240, refers to the historian Xanthus of Sardis. Athenaeus has a full account of his madness: "Cambles was a hearty eater and a hearty drinker, even a glutton." When he awoke to find his wife's hand in his mouth, he cut his throat: Athenaeus, *Deipnosophistae*, 10.15 (4:3381); Tixier, *Officina*, 5.51 (811).

[14] Villafranca: probably Villafranca da Forlì, just a few miles from Garzoni's birthplace.

Pietro Antonio from Val di Taro, a gardener by profession, did a more serious thing: discovering that some of his vegetables had been ruined during the night, he became seized with such fury and had so much rage that, using his teeth, he devoured a hoe, a shovel, and a manure wagon, unable to appease the great fury which, beyond all reason, had driven him to such insanity.

Similar to him was Domenicone of Guastalla.[15] Unfortunately, one morning he found that a bed of fava beans had been ruined, and because of this trifling matter he got into such a state of insanity that he decided never to farm again, and ate the bean-poles, the wagon, and the oxen, all in less than five days.

Let this be enough to show why—with good reason—these folks are called Furious and Beastly Madmen in Need of Ropes and Chains. They display outside their cell the god Mars[16] as their sign because he is the source of the fantastical humors which they have in their heads. Therefore let us have recourse to that god who stokes the fire of their insanity, so that it will be stirred as little as possible, returning them to their former selves, relieved of their folly.

An Oration to the God Mars, On Behalf of Violent, Beastly Madmen in Need of Ropes and Chains

To you, eldest son of Jupiter and Juno, sometimes called Mars, sometimes Mamertus, and other times Mavors, because you turn weighty matters upside-down, now Mars Ultor, now God Gradivius, dear Brother-in-Law to the goddess Bellona,[17] I come to commend to you these Violent and Beastly Madmen, who are continually growing in their foolish temperament, so that by withdrawing your ferocious influence from their heads, they will let themselves be tied up like little lambs, just as you were tied up together with Venus in Vulcan's net.[18] So if, in addition to the songs of the Salian priests,[19] you desire to hear a bagpipe in your temple and, in addition to the wolf and the green woodpecker[20] which were offered to you in ancient times, you wish to see the paw of a great beast consecrated to you, give some hope for health to these miserable creatures, who will not fail to offer to you as much as they have promised.

---

[15] Guastalla: on the Po, about 30 miles south of Mantua.

[16] Mars' attributes and epithets are in Giraldi, *De deis gentium*, 10 (313–320).

[17] Bellona, Mars' sister, goddess of war.

[18] Initially woven by Vulcan to capture Mars and Venus (see Brumble, *Myths*, 207–9), this magic net reappears in *Orlando Furioso*, where the monster Caligorante tries to capture Astolfo in it. Instead, the monster himself becomes caught in it.

[19] Salian priests: members of a Roman cult dedicated to Mars. They would sing and dance ("Salian" means "dancers").

[20] Green woodpecker: a bird sacred to Mars.

The Twenty-Fifth Discourse: The Over-the-Top and Triple-Refined

It is usual and customary to name certain men in the world by the title of Over-the Top or Triple-refined Madmen[1] when they possess certain sort of joviality which tends toward the extreme. Or they possess a certain rashness and unusual daring which incites them to say and do certain extreme things that bear a similarity to the temperament they possess. These people are for the most part vain, and most of them tend toward buffoonery, telling jokes to make people laugh and doing zany things with no regard for the time. In fact, even if it is Lent, they put Carnival back on its feet, and whether it is a day of fasting or one of feasting, they are always in the mood to do crazy things, without regard—I would say—to the time nor the place nor the people nor a thousand other important circumstances.

The ancient example of Damasippius of Athens, celebrated by Celio, can show us in what way he was an outstanding Over-the Top or Triple-refined Fool.[2] He was so well-preserved in this material that—being always merry—he could hold forth in front of anyone, like a little joker. Partly with ape-like moves, partly with monkey-smiles, partly with witticisms, partly with sayings and other babble, he entertained his audience for many hours, sometimes playing dissolutely with those who slapped him in the face, responding with a few well-chosen quips.

One could say that in our day Antonello da Rubia is to be counted among the ranks of these Over-the-Top Madmen, because you could always find him in a mood like this, so that it seemed that he had a hornet's nest that incited him to perform comedies and gigs. Among other episodes, this one is remarkable: once, he was in the presence of a lord of some importance and, falling into a skip-and-a-jump with usual foolery, made so many different faces, mimicked so well some fools of his hometown, and went so seriously into all sorts of buffoonery that the lord came close to dying from laughter.

---

[1] "Triple-refined," or *tre cotte*, typically said of sugar, to indicate in this case a very high-quality fool. Cf also p. 51, note 42.

[2] Damasippius: famous mime and comic also known as Caligula; his anecdote is not found in Celio, but both Cherchi and Fiorato agree that the anecdote came from Juvenal, *Satires*, 8.185. Damasippius is also the subject of an adage, *Insania non omnibus eadem*, in Erasmus, *Adages*, 3.10.97.

The man who was called the Emperor of Bologna—although he is not well known by all—was full of this same light wine.[3] Among his other feats, this wonderful one is told by those who knew him: one day he was appointed to substitute for a certain judge who had left him in charge of making certain public pronouncements in his absence—ones that were flatly against the freedom of the people and against his own too, and for this reason were despised by all factions. But like the Over-the-Top Madman that he was, he himself played the bugler. After he had made them public, he said that the judge was having a good time, and that he had served him by making them public. But anyone who wanted to observe them could do so if they wished, but as for him, he was not willing to observe any of them. He left the entire world with great laughter, as they sensed the great affection that he had for those proclamations.

The other one, called Donkey's Jaw by the common people, was, just like the previous one, certainly one of this tribe too. He was in the service of a very rich Spanish cavalier who one day threatened to *tomarle* or take off his *cabeza*. Feigning not to understand him—even though he understood very well—he went to the stable where there were ten or twelve *cavezze* or harnesses for the horses and, bringing them to his master, he said that his Illustrious Master could *tomasse* or take any of them that he wanted, but he would certainly want to leave the one on his *valigione* or pack-horse.[4] At this, the Spaniard was forced to laugh at his joke, and, getting over his anger, he took him back into his previous graces.

The ones who are similar to these therefore are called Over-the-Top or Triple-refined Madmen, and they have in front of their cell in our Hospital the image of the goddess Volupia or Voluptina[5] —so devoutly revered by the Romans—whom we invoke to assist them, according to our custom, with the following oration:

---

[3] "Full . . . . wine," having the same characteristics as the previous example.

[4] The story plays on "removing a harness" versus "taking his head off." There is also a play on "valligiano," or valley-dweller, and "valigione," or pack-horse, a reference to Mascella himself.

[5] Voluptina: Roman goddess of pleasure: Giraldi, *De deis gentium*, 1:49.

An Oration to the Goddess Voluptina, on Behalf of Excessive and Triple-refined Madmen

For the many entertainments and for the many pleasures that are held within your dear breast, O Goddess Voluptina! For the laughter of Democritus![6] For that of Philistion of Nicaea,[7] who burst from laughing! For the bliss of the comic Philippides[8] who died of joy! For the joy of Lacedemonian Cheilon,[9] who died in the loving embrace of his son, crowned at Olympia! For the many giggles which ever escaped from the mouth of the god Liber![10] For all of the gaiety that one finds in the entire choir of Graces! I pray and pray once more, and then return to pray again, that you will restrain as much as possible the violent disposition of these Over-the-Top Fools toward boasting and joy, so that, even if they are not cured, at least they will be improved through your favor and intercession. And if you do so, you can be certain that they will hang one of those cymbals good for singing "In the Merry, Merry Month of May,"[11] as a sign that, with such loving succor, you have joyfully relieved these miserable souls. Remain in peace, dear child.[12]

---

[6] Democritus, the "laughing philosopher."

[7] Philistion of Nicaea: famous comic at the time of Tiberius; he is credited with having restored Greek mime: Tixier, *Officina*, 2.87 (238). See Smith, *Dictionary of Greek and Roman Biography*, "Philistion": 3.294.

[8] Philippides: comic Greek poet (fourth to third centuries B.C.), member of the "new comedy" movement. Philippides died of joy when, at an advanced age, he unexpectedly won a poetry contest: Aulus Gellius, *Attic Nights*, 3.15 (1: 285).

[9] Cheilon: politician and Spartan hero, considered one of the seven wise men of Greece. He died of joy after his son won a prize at the Olympics. All of these examples of fatal laughter are in Tixier, *Officina*, 2.87, "Of Joyful and Morbid Laughter" (238).

[10] See p. 74, note 18.

[11] The first line of a famous ballad by Angelo Poliziano, *Poesie italiane*, intro. Mario Luzi. ed. Salverio Orlando (Milan: Rizzoli, 1998), 143.

[12] The last phrase is somewhat obscure. Cherchi suggests that the orignial "*fia*" should be "*sia*," while Barelli argues that "*fia*" is correct and is a regional form of "child." We adopt this second reading here.

The Twenty-Sixth Discourse: The Obstinate, Like a Mule

That breed of Marche donkeys full of such obstinacy—they seem to be harder than diamonds and you must plead with them for four hours just to get them to do the smallest part of what they are supposed to do, being haughty by nature and stiff as a rod—are, in our Hospital of Madmen, properly termed Madmen as Obstinate as a Mule.

In the Holy Scriptures, the stubborn Pharaoh was a most notable example of one of these.[1] His marble bust left a sad legacy of one who was a most obstinate fool, so that one might wonder whether he was the son of Obstinacy herself, or whether he was, in fact, her father and progenitor.

Another fool of this type was depicted by the ecclesiastical writers, namely, Julian the Apostate, who was, during his lifetime, always the adversary and enemy of Christ.[2] Even while his wicked and accursed soul was exhaling for the last time, he did not repent his contemptuousness, but, insane with anger and rage toward Him, even though he did confess to having been defeated, he tried to find words full of contempt for the Victor, and said, "Galilean, You have won!"

All of the cruel tyrants of antiquity such as Dionysius, Busiris, Phalaris, Hieronymus, Policrates, Creon,[3] and the more modern ones, such as Ezzelino da Romano,[4]

---

[1] Exodus 7–12.

[2] Julian the Apostate (A.D. 331–363), politician, philosopher, and Roman general. After usurping the emperorship, he renounced Christianity and adopted the cult of Mithra, then persecuted Christians and promoted the ancient pagan religions. According to tradition, at the moment of his death, he is said to have cried out, "Galilean, you have won!" See Jacobus de Voragine, *The Golden Legend: Readings on the Saints*, trans. Ryan, 2:135–37.

[3] Garzoni invokes some of the most infamous tyrants of antiquity: Dionysius of Syracuse; Busiris, king of Egypt, who put to death all foreigners (see also p. 180); Phalaris, tyrant of Agrigento, who burned at the stake his human victims; Hieronymus, king of Syracuse; Polycrates, tyrant of Samos; Creon, tyrant of Thebes who killed members of his own family, Polynice, Antigone, and Haemon. Tixier, *Officina*, 3.2, "Of Tyrants" (293).

[4] Ezzelino da Romano III, called The Tyrant (d. 1359). For a selection of modern research on this figure, see Giorgio Cracco, ed., *Nuovi studi ezzeliniani*, 2 vols. (Rome: Istituto Palazzo Borromini, 1992).

Valentino,⁵ and others, are assigned to this infamous and vituperative gang, not to mention that vile bunch of those whose folly would never have been recorded by writers had I not put them in this Hospital—which was built to incarcerate them.

Among those I will mention is one who would make a man hit his head against a wall because of the annoyance caused by so much asinine, mulish obstinacy, as we wish to call it. It was found in a man who was worthy of being flogged with a stick—just as they knock walnuts out of the trees—whose name was Bronte of Santo Alberto.⁶ He was born to be a spectacular example of remarkable rigidity and an obstinate mind. One day he firmly proposed that where Donatus says *Ianua sum rudibus*,⁷ "Ianua" in this case meant "Genoa" and cited a medical dictionary by a Mister Simone from Genoa⁸ who had compiled all of Galen's works, where he said he had seen it used this way. And even though there was no lack of learned men of letters who, noting this buffoonery, openly argued with him over his obstinate position, this Apulian jackass refused to change his mind and accept that it meant "the door." He would reply again and again, first with one argument, then with another, until, finally, being determined not to humiliate himself by giving in, he said that if it didn't mean "Genoa" it also didn't mean "door," but did mean "porter." Then, noting the subtlety of the buffoon who had argued so logically, everyone crossed themselves because it was a miracle that he had conceded so much to the honorable congregation around him.

Another arch-pedant, a most pedantic of pedants—for this is the most hard-headed breed, being the most ignorant in the world—was called The Lisper. One day he happened to get into a debate with the schoolmaster, a well-educated, intelligent man, graced with excellent manners. They argued over the words of Cato, *Troco lude, aleas fuge*⁹ or "Play with the hoop, avoid the dice." With much obstinacy, he maintained that in this saying Cato had given permission to children to play pool,¹⁰ and that in their diets they should always avoid garlic sauce.¹¹ He maintained this with such vehemence that the teacher, clever and well-advised, left him in his ignorance and said that he was right. The inculcated pedagogue, still obstinate, said, "Now you see that I

---

⁵ Valentino: Caesare Borgia, Duke of Valentino (1475–1507), famous tyrant. See Machiavelli, *The Prince*, 7.

⁶ Santo Alberto: possibly the town 20 miles north of Venice.

⁷ *Ianua sum rudibus*: "I am the door for the ignorant," first line of a grammatical saying very well-known at the end of the Middle Ages: Fiorato, n. 631.

⁸ Simon of Genoa, Simon Genuensis: compiler of the works of Galen and author of a medical text, *Clavis sanationis* (1473).

⁹ Cato, *Disticha Catonis*, Prologus, 36.

¹⁰ Troco or troco: a game played with a hoop and dice. Trucco: a game similar to billiards. Barelli, 145, notes 14 and 15.

¹¹ A play on "*aleas*," Latin for "dice," and "*aglio*," Italian for "garlic."

knew what I was saying, because I have read Diomedes[12] and Scopa[13] and Priscanese[14] more than four times and I have a dictionary entitled *Tortellio Novarese*[15] which will set straight anyone who wishes to persist in arguing with me."

Enough about these fools who are called Obstinate like Mules. In our Hospital they maintain for their devotions the image of Minos,[16] a divinity truly appropriate to them. So with solemn prayers, let us have recourse to his favor which is most appropriate and beneficial to them.

An Oration to the God Minos on Behalf of the Obstinate, like Mules

O Severe above All Severe Ones, Inexorable, Merciless, Unmovable, Inflexible god of the Stygian Lake, natural son of Jupiter and Europa, Most Mighty King of Crete, husband of that Pasiphaë who, because of her lust, fell in love with a bull and shamefully slept with him; Bitter Persecutor of Daedalus because he built that wooden cow in which your libidinous wife hid and where she had the opportunity for that dishonest intercourse with him.[17] By that hard and rigid severity which everybody attributes to you, both in this as well as all the other foolish acts attributed to you, I pray, beseech, and implore you that with these obstinate ones—who have taken your image for their devotions—you will proceed in such a way that they—uncautious ones!—may realize that their obstinacy is very different from yours. Yes, different: because you were always unbending in fair and honest matters, while they have hammered the nail so firmly into unjust and truly unseemly things that one cannot discern any similarity between your nature and theirs. Therefore, O Most Holy Deity of the Kingdom of Dis, make known the difference between you and them, and offer them that obstinacy that reigns in you. Because of the grace that you will show to this obstinate gang, you will see offered to you as your reward a gigantic heel like the ones the peasants of Romagna put on their shoes. It will be nailed up in front of your image as a sign and will indicate that the rigidity that they pray to you for has a different utility than theirs.

---

[12] Diomedes: Latin grammarian of the fourth century A.D., author of an *Ars grammatica* used by students.

[13] Scopa: Lucio Giovani Scopa, philologist active at the beginning of the sixteenth century, author of the *Grammatices institutiones* (Naples, 1521).

[14] Francesco Priscianese, Florentine author of a *Dictionarium ciceronianum* and of the textbook *De' principi de la lengua romana* (1540).

[15] *Tortellio Novarese*: a reference to Giovanni Tortelli d'Arezzo's *Commentarium de orthographia dictionum ex graecis tractarum* (Rome, 1471).

[16] Minos: a semi-mythic hero, king and legislator from Crete. Dante assigns him the role of a judge in the Inferno because of his severity. See Brumble, *Myths*, 222–23.

[17] These attributes are in Giraldi, *De deis gentium*, 7 (216).

The Twenty-Seventh Discourse: The Hairless

Those who enjoy annoying and irritating first one person, then another, are commonly called Hairless Madmen.[1] They are unable to restrain their humor, but are constantly silly toward first one, then another, causing this to happen: that most or even all people—or at least the most important—join together and, taking vengeance against them, make them remain Hairless Fools. In fact, these are the ones who accumulate blows[2] and take home wallops which they frequently deserve for their asinine importunities. The less they think about it (because they overestimate their worth[3] and their intelligence, they ride at full gallop, confident that they can outdo their companions in all things—since they consider others to be of no more importance than a tavern sign), the more they are caught being at fault. It is rare that he who is very presumptuous about himself does not get his comeuppance from someone who stands into the wind,[4] on guard to fool the very person who is trying to fool him.

Catiline[5] thought that he could outsmart Cicero in the grand plot he had devised against him. But this wise and quick-witted man called down the entire brigade onto his head. With the help of that woman,[6] Cicero uncovered his dealings, and trapped him in such a way that finally, according to what Sallust writes, he, together with all of his accomplices, ended up like Hairless Fools.

Ludovico, called Il Moro, according to Guicciardini,[7] thought that he would play a trick on Ferdinand, king of Naples, by calling the French into Italy against

---

[1] "Hairless," having lost their hair by constantly butting into other people.

[2] Collect bumps and bruises.

[3] The original has *huomo*, or man. Barelli (147, n. 3) believes that "*buono*" or "worth" is correct.

[4] "stand into the wind," *sta all'orza:* an idiom meaning to stand guard.

[5] Catiline (108–62 B.C.), recounted by Sallust in *The War with Catiline*. His deceitful acts were denounced by Cicero in the Roman Senate in his vehement *Catilinarians*.

[6] "that woman": Fulvia, the lover of Quintus Curius, a co-conspirator with Catiline. Fulvia exposed the conspiracy as described by Sallust, *The War with Catiline*, 23.3.

[7] Francesco Guicciardini, *Storia d'Italia*, 15:6.

him.⁸ But in the end, something that the Florentine ambassador had figured out about him turned out to be true—he had seen his coat-of-arms in Milan (which showed a Moor sweeping up garbage from in front of a lady),⁹ and expressed his opinion, namely that Il Moro should watch out because, by sweeping up the trash, he would draw it to himself. In fact, in the end he wound up a Hairless Fool, losing his country, his life, and his honor all at the same time.¹⁰

Similarly, Lorenzino de' Medici, a very close relative of Duke Alessandro I, thought that he would perform a heroic deed by treacherously murdering the Duke in a room in his palace—as Giovio¹¹ tells us and, more extensively, Ruscelli.¹² Nothing fell on him for this misdeed other than that because of it he became infamous as a traitor to the whole world, and transformed peaceful happiness into perpetual agitation of both body and soul. Finally, in keeping with his merits, he was murdered in Venice by someone else's men.¹³

And this? Didn't that Bourbon¹⁴—so widely known for the sack of Rome—think that he could deal a marvelous blow when he suddenly turned on his king who, in his courtesy, magnanimity, and all sorts of other virtues, will always have no peer? Whereas in the end everyone considered him an infamous traitor. And, as Bugati reported, he provided an occasion for that Castilian gentleman with the most generous soul to demonstrate his innate greatness

---

⁸ Ludovico Il Moro, Duke of Milan, put out an appeal to Charles VIII (1494) to intervene in Italy to consolidate his holdings and defeat the king of Naples, Ferdinand II. This campaign marked the beginning of the Italian wars. See Guicciardini, *Storia d'Italia*, I, 4, 6–11; Fiorato, n. 658.

⁹ The anecdote is told in Paolo Giovio's *Trattato delle imprese*, 44. The Florentine ambassador is Francesco Gualtierotti.

¹⁰ During the second French campaign (1499–1500), Ludovico Il Moro was in effect defeated, robbed of his estates, and taken prisoner to France, where he died in 1513. Garzoni's criticism of Ludovico reflects the widespread Italian opinion that he had committed treason and received just punishment, since he was considered responsible for Italy's defeat: Fiorito, n. 659.

¹¹ Paolo Giovio's *Historiarum sui temporis libri II* (Florence: Torrentini, 1550–1552).

¹² Girolamo Ruscelli, *Sopplimento di Girolamo Ruscelli nell'Historie di Monsignor Paolo Giovio* (Venice: Silicato, 1572), 30–37.

¹³ The assassination of the first Duke of Florence, Alessandro de' Medici, by his cousin Lorenzino was carried out in 1537. Lorenzino was murdered in 1548.

¹⁴ "That Bourbon" is Duke Charles de Bourbon, commander of the Bourbon forces who died during the sack of Rome in 1527, falling from a ladder while he was attempting to scale the walls of the city. He is said to have been killed by Benvenuto Cellini. The king against whom he turned is Charles VIII. Garzoni works several disparate stories into his account: his opinion that the king was responsible for the sack of Rome; an elegy to the "Most Christian" King; and his account, according to the historian Gasparo Bugati, of an anecdote which highlights the infamy of the commander: Fiorito, n. 662.

and Castilian pride to Charles the Fifth. For when that emperor asked him, as a favor, to lend him his palace to provide lodging for the Bourbon, he said that it would not be possible for him to deny anything to His Sacred Majesty, but he was certain that when the Bourbon left, he would destroy the palace right down to its foundations so that no one could say or point out that "This is the palace of such-and-such a gentleman where the Bourbon traitor stayed."

Didn't Giorgio Sanese[15] also think that he could accomplish a wonderful blow when he wanted to deliver the castle of Milan into the hands of the French? And when his act of treason was discovered, the traitor lost Luna's friendship, his own life, and his reputation all at the same time.

And didn't the French Huguenots think—as Tasso wrote[16]—that they could carry off a brilliant act when they assembled in Paris for the marriage of the king's sister[17] with Navarre,[18] conspiring to kill off the royal house and to ruin Paris? And they certainly ended up Hairless Fools in the end because the Admiral,[19] with all of his sect, had the upper hand because of their memory of Charles IX and from the lords who were his followers, and who knew much more about it than all of them together.

All of these therefore are called Hairless Fools with good reason, because in the end they are caught just as they think that they have fooled others. They have for their sign in our Hospital, a Rhadamanthus[20] to whom I turn to ask for help, as usual—with sword drawn—for these miserable, ignorant and comical sorts.

An Oration to Rhadamanthus on Behalf of the Hairless

There is not one among all of the judges who is more just or more severe than you and Minos, together with Aeacus, son of Aegina and Jupiter. For this reason you who, in the Kingdom of Dis,[21] serve in the highest post are deservedly called upon to heal

---

[15] Giorgio Sanese: a military officer who offered to deliver the castle of Milan to the French, an enterprise that was blocked by Juan de Luna, governor of Milan at the time. See Gasparo Bugati, *Historia universale* (Venice: Giolito, 1571), Book 7 (970): Cherchi, 345.

[16] "Tasso": Faustino Tasso, in *Le historie dei successi de' nostri tempi* (Venice: Guerra, 1583). Beretti, 149, n. 16.

[17] Margaret of Valois.

[18] Henry of Navarre, the future Henry IV.

[19] The Admiral: Gaspard de Coligny, who was one of the first victims of the massacre: Fiorato, n. 666. He was a subject of the famous "defenestration."

[20] Rhadamanthus: Cretan hero, famous for his justice and political wisdom. Because of this he was called to Hell to judge the dead with his brothers, Minos and Aeacus (Brumble, *Myths*, 222). He is the subject of two Erasmian adages: 2.9.30 and 31 (34:101–2).

[21] "Kingdom of Dis": Hades.

this sort of most unjust fool. Therefore, I pray to you, do what is expected of your duty and we will offer to you a worn-out gown, kept in the hands of a Jew for more than ten years—and which certainly has no nap left on it—as testimony to the whole world that there is no one who is better at keeping the upper hand over these Hairless Madmen—subjects to that whip which miraculously chastens their sort.

The Twenty-Eighth Discourse: The Unbridled, Like a Horse

The overly unrestrained behave excessively and recklessly, and they usurp the freedom to offend others—either with words or deeds—because they assume that the entire world is theirs. And they assume that they can run up against anyone, at their pleasure, with their abused freedom. These are termed, in a word, Unbridled Madmen Like Horses since they have an indomitable mind and an excessively outspoken nature inside them. And with no other epithet would I be able to describe with greater ease the qualities of this foolish gang who kick with their hooves—straight on or cross-wise—anyone they meet.

It seems that Seneca, in his *Epistles*, places a certain Oscus in their number. It is said that he was born into the world never to be at peace, but instead to be always restless, bothering first this person and then that one with his words and deeds all day long.[1]

And, in a few words, the poets have included Momus[2] among these men, for he was so petulant that these words were written about him:

Nullum opus tam absolutum esse poterat, quod non calumniaretur Momus.

It was not possible to create a work so perfect that Momus would not speak badly of it.

---

[1] Oscus or frequently, Moschus: Seneca, *Controversiae*, 10, Preface, 10. Also in Manuzio, *Adagia* (855). See Garzoni, *Piazza*, ed. Cherchi and Collina, 30 n. 6. Garzoni's source is undoubtedly Tixier, *Officina*, 5.38, "On Free and Importune Loquacity" (777–79).

[2] Momus was the personification of mockery and censure: Hesiod, *Theogony*, 214, quoted in Tixier, *Officina*, 5.38 (778). Garzoni's source was most likely the comic work *Momus* by Leon Battista Alberti, written in 1450, in which his anti-hero lambastes various of his contemporaries, including the pope. See *Momus*, ed. and trans. Sarah Knight (Cambridge, MA: Harvard University Press, 2004). Momus also appears in the prologue of Garzoni's *Piazza*.

A very ridiculous occurrence suffices as evidence of this condition. One day, looking at that beautiful Venus sculpted by the divine Pheidias,[3] he had to at least say this: that the buckle on her shoe was not done very well. These are the men who, because of their ill-affected nature, are always looking for a hair in their egg. [4]

In our time, Marinello da Gambacorta[5] was one of these unbridled fools. It happened that one time he had the opportunity to attend a performance in Vicenza, and he began to say bad things during the Prologue and continued through all the acts, saying bad things just for the sake of argument, about this and that comic actor, to the point that a man who was sitting near him was driven by his irritation to say, "Dear fellow, take off your overcoat, then we will gladly hear the Arch-Beast speak his lines." [6]

Another example, not unlike the preceding one, is that of the man from Porcia who had the nickname Horse's Halter, because he needed nothing as much as he needed a horse's halter. A friend took him to see the hall of the Grand Council of Venice when it was full of many gentlemen and nobles, all truly resplendent with their magnificent physical bearing and their air of grave majesty befitting the grand senators that they were.[7] Like the clumsy elephant he was, he began to make comments—no less insensibly than ridiculously—on this man's hat, that man's nose, how that man stood, and how that other one walked. He didn't leave this spectacle—certainly the great honor and adornment, not only of Italy but of all Christendom—until he had gone through almost the entire list of this most honorable gathering. Then, a perceptive senator near him gestured with his glove for the man to approach him and had the man come before him. The senator asked him where he was from, and, having learned that he was from Porcia[8] and knowing from his name that his nickname was Horse's Halter, he grabbed him by his collar[9] and said, "Sir Grunt from Porcia, how good it would be for you to wear a halter! But, if you please, return to Porcia unless you want to be turned into a pork chop." Burned by and crestfallen at these words, he turned to his friend and said, "For God's sake, let's get out of here, because that gentleman

---

[3] Pheidias (490–431 B.C.), the most famous Athenian sculptor. Fiorato indicates that Garzoni is referring to one of two lost works described by Pausanias (*Description of Greece*, 1.14.7 and 6.25.1); one, the Aphrodite Urania, planned for Elis, the second, the Aphrodite of Paros marble sculpted for a sanctuary in Athens: Fiorato, n. 678. See p. 38, note 14.

[4] "Hair in their egg": looking for the smallest imperfection.

[5] Gambacorta: an unidentified town, but literally "short-legged," hence defective.

[6] "take off your overcoat," meaning "get ready to act the part of the fool that you are."

[7] Such orations before the Venetian Senate was an obligatory topos in the letters of the sixteenth century: Fiorato, n. 679.

[8] Porcia or Porzia: small town near Pordenone, about 40 miles northeast of Venice. Also a play on *porca*, "sow."

[9] *Cavezzo* means "halter," "collar," and "hangman's noose."

whom you saw whispered in my ear that there is a penalty of three pulls on the cord[10] for anyone who stands at this gate!"

In our time, this type of fool is represented by Aretino, Franco, Burchiello, Bernia,[11] and other similar friends of Pasquino and Marforio.[12] So it is no wonder that they have been overcome and restrained with a halter by those against whom they proved to be so dissolute and slobbery beyond measure. Nor is anything else appropriate for fools such as these but a good halter to gag their throats in such a way that they cannot vomit up that awful *Amarulentia* or bitterness that they hold inside themselves with such difficulty.[13]

So these Unbridled Fools or Fools like a Horse keep the image of Hippona[14] in front of their cell in our Hospital, as the proper goddess for their needs. Therefore, with the following oration, we will try to placate her in such a way that she will not allow these ferocious and cursed beasts to kick so much with their hooves.

An Oration to the Goddess Hippona on Behalf of the Unbridled

O Goddess of the Dungheap, when the ancients assigned your agreeable image to stables, this was done not out of disrespect, but because they knew that all animals have their favorite god or deity, just as Sylvanus is the god of sheep,[15] Miagrus is the god of flies, and Bubona is the goddess of oxen.[16] Likewise, you were adored as the goddess who protects horses and their stables. If Nicolò, the coachman for the Santi Quaranta,[17] knew about this, you can be certain that—even though he is a poor man—he would not think it an imposition to spend four

---

[10] "Pulls on the cord": tightens the rack on which victims were tortured. Our madman fabricates a face-saving excuse for having to depart so quickly.

[11] With this grouping of these famous authors with "fools of this type," Garzoni criticizes the major satirical and anti-conformist poets of the fifteenth and sixteenth centuries—all very harsh critics of cultural standards and societal norms. Burchiello (1404–1448), Aretino (1492–1557), Niccolò Franco (1515–1570), and Francesco Berni (1497–1535) "had trouble with the censors": Fiorato, n. 689.

[12] "Pasquino and Marforio": statues to which the Romans would attach satires and epigrams. See Fiorato, n. 690.

[13] *Amarulentia*: the word evokes Romans 3:14, *Quorum os execratione et amarulentia plenum*, "Their mouths are full of cursing and bitterness."

[14] "Hippona," goddess of horses and manure: Giraldi, *De deis gentium*, I.46.

[15] "Sylvan," also god of forests, mountains, and fields.

[16] These three gods are treated in Giraldi, *De deis gentium*, 1.46.

[17] Santi Quaranta: a title of the Cardinals of Saranda in Albania.

bezzi[18] to purchase your image to tack up on the poop-deck of his carriage so that you would be the protectress of his horses forever.

So for this reason, these worthless draft-horses may be commended to you, so that, were they good for nothing else, at least they will be able to fill up three or four basins.

If, as usual, you benignly look at their needs with your pitiful eyes, you will see that very quickly you will be made an offering of something other than empty words, because when you least expect it, you will find in front of your image a couple of giant saddle-bags like those of Gonella,[19] by which one will know that these men are now loaded down with insults whereas previously they were unbridled and no restraint was good enough to keep them in check.

---

[18] *bezzi*: Venetian coins.
[19] Gonella, see p. 147, note 14..

The Twenty-Ninth Discourse: The Extravagant, Extreme, and Witless

Madmen who do certain extravagantly foolish things, peculiar and novel, which far surpass the bounds of the usual, things which are not known to be performed by others, are given the common terms Extravagant, Extreme, and Witless.

Aelian[1] reported on a certain Thrasyllos of Axione who fell into this amazing folly: he believed that all of the ships that arrived at the port were his own, so that before they had arrived at the dock he would go to meet them with a countenance and heart full of joy and contentment. And similarly, when they sailed away on a voyage to the East or to the West, he would accompany them a good piece of the way, wishing them well with a good heart, fair winds and a prosperous voyage.

Aristotle also tells of a man from Abydos[2] who, beginning to go crazy, and continuing in that state for many days, would go to the theater and, as if he wanted to act in a comedy, he would make all those gestures which comics ordinarily use on stage.

Plutarch tells the tragic story of certain maidens from Miletus who were assailed by such great insanity that, without thinking, they all hung themselves. Neither the memory of their elders nor the tears of their fathers and mothers could help retrieve them from their insanity. Finally, as the Milesians were assembled in their senate, debating this matter, one of their most brilliant men arose and said that if these women persisted with this sort of silly thinking, it would be necessary to pass a law that they would all be stripped and left hanging naked and displayed in public. When this decree was approved by all and subsequently implemented, it put the girls into such a state of terror that they restrained themselves from their inclination, because as free women, honesty was stronger in them than insanity.[3]

---

[1] *Historiae variae*, 4.25. Aelian goes on to tell that Thrasyllos' brother took him to a healer who cured him of his ailment. However, in reflecting on his life, he said that he never enjoyed life more than when he was looking after his ships.

[2] Abydos: town in Mysia, on the Hellespont. The story is in Pseudo-Aristotle, *Mirabilia*, 31.892b.

[3] This anecdote, describing their love-sickness which led to their suicide, was reported by Aulus Gellius, *Attic Nights*, 15.10. It was repeated a number of times by ancients

Similar to the deaths of these women was the end of Laurenziano from Florence, a most learned man, and of Leonio, a brilliant philosopher in his own time. According to Pietro Crinito,[4] both of them, without any reason or misfortune whatsoever, threw themselves down a well where, no less foolishly than miserably, they ended their days.[5]

A truly extreme case of madness was that of Teobaldo da Cantiana.[6] He was convinced that he was the Sultan of Egypt, and would frequently go barefoot and with a turban on his head into a certain cave near his hometown which he called the Great Mosque. He would bring a litter of piglets with him to the entrance of the cave, saying that they were the ambassadors of princes who were accompanying him to honor him. When he entered the cave, he would make the cave resound with these verses which he sang:

> Listen, Mohammedans, to what Teobaldo,
> Who is now The Great Sultan, has to say:
> If you don't study the Koran
> None of you will die happy.

Another one, called Scarpaccia of Gradisca,[7] had an extravagant humor in his head, we might say, because he got the idea that he was the King of Cuckoos[8] and he would always reply to everyone who spoke to him—regardless of whether it was good or bad—by saying "cuckoo, cuckoo, cuckoo," three times. When asked why he didn't respond in a sensible way, he would again reply "I am the King, cuckoo, cuckoo, cuckoo."

I remember having heard it said that a certain Alberto from Pietra Mala—which is on the border of the territory of Bologna—was definitely one of these extravagant ones. He entered into the fantasy that he had become the Lord of Mirandola and wrote a letter to the citizens of that town saying that they should turn over their castle to him. When he received no response to his

---

such as Plutarch, "The Bravery of Women," 11, *Moralia* 249b-d, and by contemporaries of Garzoni like Bandello: Fiorato, n. 705; also in Tixier, *Officina* 2.98 (267). Garzoni writes that "they all hung themselves," but that is not true. This is Garzoni's only example of madness in women included in the sections of *The Hospital* otherwise devoted to men. Since this example of female madness appears in proximity to the next two examples, in Tixier, *Officina* 2.98, Garzoni may have chosen to mine Tixier here at the expense of his otherwise strictly separate treatment of women.

[4] "Pietro Crinito": Pietro Riccio (1465–1507), Florentine poet and humanist, author of *De honesta disciplina;* Fiorato, n. 706.

[5] Both examples are in Tixier, *Officina* 2.98 (298).

[6] "Cantiana": Cantiano, a town north of Gubbio in Umbria.

[7] Grandisca, a small town between Pordenone and Udine.

[8] "Cuckoo": another name for a madman in Italian, as it is in English. Cf. above, p. 41, note 1; p. 43; p. 94, note 5; and p. 154, notes 7 and 8.

foolishness, he leaped onto his high-spirited horse and, putting a drum over his shoulder, he went from Pietra Mala to the outskirts of Mirandola[9] to summon them to fight with him. Then, since he was scorned for his madness once again, he went to the town wall and, answering the call of nature at the gate, he said that if the people of Mirandola didn't want him as their lord, they could at least accept this other gift that he left at their feet.

These are the fools who have in our Hospital the sign of Hercules, [10] who undoubtedly is the defender and protector for life of this species of fool. So with the oration that follows, we present this encomium to him, as is our usual practice.

An Oration to the God Hercules on Behalf of Extremely and Truly Extravagant Madmen

You are that robust and valorous son of Jupiter and Alcmene, who are called Tirynthius, because you were raised at Tiryns in Greece; and called the Theban god, because you were worshipped in Thebes; and called the god Vagus, because you wandered around conquering monsters; and called the Great Alcides, because you were a nephew of the famous Alcaeus.

You are also the one who was truly envied by Juno, because of your strength and because of the mother who bore you. Being exposed to insurmountable labors,[11] you first wore her out with your obedience before she wore herself out with demands. You are also the one who, while lying in your cradle, killed two snakes which she had put there to poison you. You are also the one who, although still a youth, was handsomely potent, and in one night impregnated fifty daughters of Thespius by whom you had fifty sons called the Thespiades. You are also the one who, as an adult, repressed the great Hydra with her seven continually-regrowing heads using both a torch and a sword near the swamp of Lernea; and you are the one who captured and killed the hind, Eripides—who looked

---

[9] Pietramala: a village in the Apennines between Bologna and Florence; Mirandola, Emilian town north of Modena.

[10] Garzoni has already mentioned Hercules as an example of a "violent, beastly" madman (Discourse XXIV). Here he is discussed in a comic manner as a mad god, a symbol of excess. His list of epithets and attributes is taken from Giraldi, *De deis gentium*, 2.324–34.

[11] Here begins a recital of the great Labors of Hercules, portrayed by Garzoni as examples of extravagant and excessive foolishness. Hercules' labors are detailed in *Herculis vita*, in Giraldi, *Opera omnia*, 2:571–598. Hercules also features prominently in Tixier, *Officina*, 2.36 (145–46). Although this long section on Hercules might seem like a digression, it should be recalled that the audience for his work prominently included the court of the Este family at Ferrara, where memories of Dukes Ercole (Hercules) d'Este I and II were still prominent. See also Brumble, *Myths*, 154–66. See also, Introduction, p. 12ff and notes.

like she was flying when she ran, with a golden horn on her head—at Mount Maenalus; and, in the Nemean forests, you slaughtered that extraordinarily large lion, and since then have always worn its pelt as a trophy; you fed Diomedes, king of Thrace, to his own horses, since he had fed them on the flesh and blood of his guests; and you captured alive and then brought back to Eurystheus that terrible wild boar on Erymanthus (a mountain in Arcadia) that was devouring everything around him.

You are also certainly the one who chased the Stymphalian birds all the way to the island of Aretias, birds so large that they obscured the sun; you tamed that bull who once ruined and destroyed with its power the entire island of Candia; you ripped off the horn of Achelous, king of Aetolia; you murdered Busiris, king of Egypt, who would devour all of the foreigners who went there; you strangled the giant Antaeus in Libya, while wrestling with him; you split up and divided Calpe and Abila[12], mountains which had previously been joined together; you held up Mount Olympus, since Atlas was tired of that great weight; you defeated in battle Geryon, king of Spain, carrying away his armor as a well-earned reward to the victor.

You are also the one who overcame the bandit Cacus, who would vomit fire from his mouth; and you murdered another one called Lacinius, who infested the outer borders of Italy, building there a temple to Juno who was therefore called Lacinia; you defeated—not far from the mouth of the Rhone River—Albion and Bergion, who were impeding the travel of first this one, then that; you defeated in battle Pyraichmes, king of Aetolia, who had made war against the Boeotians, and you chopped him up in little pieces as fine as a horse's tail.[13]

You are also the one who tamed the Centaurs; you carried the two columns to the Gades islands of Spain; you cleaned the stable of Augeas; you freed Hesione, the young daughter of Laomedon, who had been taken by a sea monster, by first killing the monster and then—aggravated because the ungrateful Laomedon declined to reward you with some good steeds which had been promised you—because of this, you destroyed the city of Troy; you sacked the island of Cos, and you killed King Eurypylus together with his children; you stripped the Amazons and made a prisoner of their queen, Hippolyte;[14] and, after descending into Hell, you tied up the three-headed Cerberus with three chains, and, thus chained up, brought him up from there.

According to many writers, you are also the one who helped Theseus abduct Proserpine, wife of Pluto; you led Alcestis, consort of King Admetus, alive out of

---

[12] Calpe and Abila, the ancient Columns of Hercules, that guard the Straits of Gibraltar.

[13] Pyraichmes: see Pausanias, *Description of Greece*, 5.4.2. This person, killed by Hercules, is not to be confused with the warrior of the Trojan War killed by Patroklos, or the hero of Elis who defeated Degmenus in a one-on-one battle.

[14] According to one tradition, Hercules killed Hippolyte to steal her girdle.

Hell and back to her husband; having returned from Hell, you killed Lycus, king of Thebes, for having raped your wife, Megara; you, with your arrows, shot the eagle that was consuming the regrown heart of Prometheus who had been bound to Mount Caucasus by Mercury; you, battling on horseback, defeated Cycnus, son of Mars, your adversary; you defeated Cecrops while serving as a maid-servant to Omphale, queen of Lydia; you destroyed Hebe with her entire household, meanwhile wounding Juno,[15] who had come to her aid; you killed Eurytus, king of Oechalia, and destroyed that city named after him.

You are also the one who took by force Iole, daughter of the above-mentioned Eurytus—who was denied to you as a wife—and took her to Euboea; you killed a serpent of immeasurable size near the river Sagaris; you slew the dragon that watched over the garden of the Hesperides; you freed the Oetans from mosquitoes and horseflies; and, finally, to produce you, it was necessary that two nights were made out of one.[16]

With all of your wonders and with all of your amazing feats, isn't it true that you can perform another labor that will seem weak and vain compared to all the others: that you, a real man, but—because of all of your extreme deeds, a god—favor these extreme fools, and get that stuff out of their heads which you drew out of the seven heads of the Hydra in one single effort? Come on now! If you do this favor for them, I promise you that, in addition to the temple which you have among the Egyptians and the Tyrians, a great chapel will be consecrated to you in this Hospital, and an oak gall[17] will be offered to you at your altar, which will serve as a sign that it is just as easy for you to free them as it is to lift up on high similar extremely light fruits[18] from among the ones we have noted.

---

[15] Juno was wounded by Hercules during the Trojan War: Homer, *Iliad*, 5.392.

[16] Hercules was conceived by Alcmene, the wife of Amphitryon, while Amphitryon was away. Zeus had disguised himself as Amphitryon and extended the night so that it was much longer than normal. During that long night, Amphitryon returned and also impregnated Alcmene. As a result, Alcmene gave birth to twin boys, Hercules and Iphicles.

[17] "oak gall" or *pan cuch*.

[18] "Light fruits," meaning, on the one hand, the oak gall, and, on the other, the vacuous, air-headed fool.

The Thirtieth Discourse: The Diabolical: Those-Deserving-of-the-Gallows-a-Thousand-Times-Over

The most brutish, bizarre, and damned sort of madmen that one can find is, without doubt, those whom we usually call by the common name of Madmen Deserving-of-the-Gallows-a-Thousand-Times-Over or Diabolical Madmen. This name is perfectly suited to their diabolical and hellish nature. They are so full of venom, so swollen with resentment, spite, and arrogance, that anyone would swear that they were true brothers of Farfarello and Calubrino.[1] Nor is there a paucity of examples of this type, for the Devil goes everywhere, sowing his seeds, like weeds,[2] and they spring forth from themselves, teeming, like the Hydra; and with the flames of their iniquity, they set fire to heaven and earth.

No one would dare deny that those giants who were struck by lightning by Jupiter for their arrogance were of this race. The author of *Etna*[3] makes this very clear with these verses:

> *Tentavere nephas olim detrudere mundo*
> *Sydera captivique Iovis transferre gigantes*
> *imperium et victo leges imponere mundo.*

> The giants—oh horrors—once tried to cause the stars to fall to earth
> and to transfer there the empire of the captive Jupiter
> and impose their laws on the defeated earth.

Similarly, it cannot be denied that Mezentius, contemptuous of the gods, was of the same race. Virgil describes him as one of them in these verses:

---

[1] "Farfarello and Calubrino": two demons of popular medieval tradition: Dante, *Inferno*, 21–22, where we find the variant, Calcabrino, who also appears in the Discourse on Women: 200 below.

[2] Matthew 13:3–28.

[3] "*Etna*," or *Aetna*, a Latin scientific poem, anonymous (but perhaps by Lucilius the Younger) of the first century A.D. It discusses the causes of volcanic eruptions, attributing them to the compression of air. The quote is from lines 43–45. Also in Tixier, *Officina*, 5.29 (753).

Primus init bellum Tyrrhenis asper ab oris
contemptor divum Mezentius.[4]

The first from Tyrrhenian lands to go to war
was that bitter despiser of the gods, Mezentius.

This is the one whom Macrobius described with these words:

Fuit impius in homines sine deorum respectu.[5]

He was impious toward men, without respect for the gods.

I consider it obvious that Lycaon, king of Arcadia, was a great Diabolical Madman, if it's true what Ovid says in the first book of his *Metamorphoses*, that he laid traps for Jupiter, who was considered by the ancients as the first god among all the gods.[6]

Nor can Xerxes, king of Persia, who was described by writers as having the greatest impiety, escape from being included in this number. He was so bold, or rather reckless, that he dared to threaten to take the sun's name away from it and to put a god of the seas into prison with shackles on his ankles. For this reason, Strozza the Elder sang about this in these verses:

Nec veluti Xerses Neptuno vincula minatur
classibus insolitum cum patefecit iter.[7]

Nor did he threaten Neptune with imprisonment, as Xerxes did, when he displayed an arrogant manner to his fleet.

Together with these fools, I place—with no second thought—that Phlegyas, King of the Lapithae and father of Ixion, who, because he had the temerity to set fire to the Delphic temple of Apollo, was punished for this offense by being banished to the caves of Hell. Virgil describes it in this way:

---

[4] *Aeneid*, 7.647–648. Mezentius was king of the Etruscans and an ally of Turnus against Aeneas, and therefore an enemy of the glorious future of Rome. Garzoni takes these examples, from the Giants to Attila and Totila, from Tixier, *Officina*, 1.18, and 5.29 and 33. Most of the examples are also to be found in Celio, *Lectiones*, 81, 361–62, 749, 1021.

[5] *Saturnalia*, 3.5.9.

[6] Ovid, *Metamorphoses*, 1.165 ff. Lycaon plotted to find out if Jupiter was a god or a man by killing him in his sleep. He next killed one of his prisoners and prepared this man to be eaten at a banquet. Jupiter caused Lycaon's house to be destroyed and him to be turned into a wolf.

[7] Father Strozza, Tito Vespasiano Strozzi; see Discourse XVIII. The quote is from *Eroticon*, 2.13–14.

>... *Phlegyasque miserrimus omnis*
> *admonet, et magna testatur voce per umbras:*
> *"Discite iustitiam moniti, et non temnere divos."*[8]

> Most wretched Phlegyas admonishes all,
> And from among the shades, he testifies:
> "Look at me and learn justice, and scorn not the gods!"

Valerius Maximus and Lactantius Firmianus[9] assign a prominent place among these sorts to Dionysius, tyrant of Syracuse, because he was such a great scorner of the gods that he himself would often say among his friends that he was really surprised that the gods were so patient that they tolerated his presence on earth for such a long time.

Biondo, in his *Histories*, told of Evarice, king of the Goths, who sealed up the doors of the Christian churches with bundles of thorns, maliciously making them appear to be thickets because he was truly a fool of this sort.[10]

Still regarding Christian churches, Corio wrote that Genseric, prince of the Vandals, with even greater sacrilege, made stables for his horses out of them, being a hellish Fool of the same type.[11]

What can we say of Attila,[12] called "The Scourge of God," if not that he was the same type? And what of Totila?[13] and what of Athanaric?[14] And what of that Duke of the Avars[15] who threatened to cut off the genitals of all the deacons who came into his hands? And what of the first who made the cathedral of Basel into a slaughterhouse for butchers?[16] And what of the many new Huguenots who

---

[8] *Aeneid*, 6.618–620. Quoted in Tixier, *Officina* 1.18 (55).

[9] Valerius Maximus, *Memorable Doings and Sayings*, 1.7. Lactantius Firmianus (d. 325–333), North African rhetorician and moralist who converted to Christianity (300 A.D). He was a tutor to Constantine's children. His works are frequently apologies for Christianity. See his *Institutiones*, 2.4 (PL 6. 272–273). The impiety of Dionysius of Syracuse was well known: Tixier, *Officina*, 1, "De deis eorumque cultu: De contemptoribus deorum" (32). Fiorato, n. 734 and Cherchi, 355, n. 8.

[10] Biondo: see 138 n. 6 above. "Evarice": king of the Goths in Spain, the son of Theodoric the First. According to historians, he was celebrated for the ravages he caused during his military campaigns in Spain, Portugal, and the south of France: Fiorato, n. 735.

[11] "Corio": see Discourse XX, 143 above. Genseric: first king of the Vandals (428–477); he is said to have exhibited the first instance of persecution by one body of Christians against another.

[12] Attila: famous king of the Huns: Tixier, *Officina*, 5.33 (769).

[13] Totila: king of the Ostrogoths (541–552): Tixier, *Officina*, 5.33 (769).

[14] Athanaric: king of the Visigoths: died 381.

[15] "the Avars" the text has "Avvi," but "Avars" seems to be meant. Originating in Central Asia, they inhabited present-day Hungary during the 6th to 8th centuries.

[16] In 1529, during a Protestant revolt, the cathedral in Basel was ravaged. According to Cherchi (356 n. 11) this may be a reference to the Council held at Basel in 1431–1449,

desperately make the worst out of anything they can, committing as many sorts of theft, violence, sacrilege, murder, and rebellion as it is possible to imagine?[17]

So these are truly the fools that deserve the gallows a thousand times over, appropriately termed Diabolical Fools because they conform to him in every detail. Therefore, in commending them to some god who can cure them, I can think of no better physician than Pluto,[18] who has a perfect cure for their kind in Hell. So I address the following oration to him to that effect:

An Oration to Pluto on Behalf of Madmen Deserving-of-the-Gallows-a-Thousand-Times-Over or Diabolical Ones

What god could I more appropriately invoke to cure the folly of these devils than you, Great Pluto, Ruler of Erebus, Master of the Stygian waves, President of those flames which exceed those of Aetna or Mongibello by a thousand times? What god, other than the one who is the son of Saturn and Ops; brother of the great Jupiter; Lord of the Infernal Kingdom; Powerful with Wealth, and therefore called Dis; First Among the Maniae[19] and therefore called Summanus, Most Powerful so as to inflict on them their due punishments and therefore called by everyone Orcus?[20] What god, if not the one who cut out Tityos' heart, punishes Tantalus with thirst, causes Ixion to be turned on the wheel, makes Sisyphus roll the stone, punishes Salmoneus with so many chastisements?[21] You, Avenger of Excesses, Revenger of Misdeeds, Beater of the Impious, Flogger of the Wicked, take care to cure these men's folly in the same way that you have cured so many. And put them into the hands of the Furies who, enraged against them, will in-

---

which led to a schism.

[17] Garzoni blames the Huguenots for the bloody religious wars being waged in his time. Earlier, in Discourse XXVII, he blames the St. Bartholemew's Day Massacre on the Huguenots.

[18] Pluto: god of the Underworld.

[19] Maniae: underworld gods, perhaps evoking the Harpies or Furies.

[20] Orcus: god of the dead, another of Pluto's appellations because of his diabolical nature. Our word "ogre" is derived from Orcus. These epithets are taken from Giraldi, who devotes ten dense pages to the gods of the Underworld (*De deis gentium*, 6 [192–203]). Orcus is the subject of an Erasmian adage: *in orci culum incidas*, "may you fall into Orcus' anus." Erasmus explains, "the words of a man who wishes someone destruction and a final end": *Adages*, 2.10.68 (34:153)

[21] Garzoni lists the major tortures of the Underworld according to Greek mythology: Tantalus, doomed to live in a lake from which he could never drink; Ixion, lashed to a flaming wheel; Sisyphus, forever to push a huge rock up a hill; Salmoneus, struck by thunderbolts because he believed himself to be the equal of the gods; and Tityos, also struck by thunderbolts and left for vultures to eat his liver. See Brumble, *Myths*, 279–81.

flict on them those torments which the seriousness of their malady deserves. If you do this soon, you will undoubtedly be offered a snail with broken antennae[22] as an illustration of the punishment you will have inflicted on them because of their shortcomings and the excesses that they have so devilishly committed.

---

[22] "snail with a broken antennae": an image of beaten-down pride in these diabolical madmen.

On Madness in Women[1]

A Discourse by the Author to the Spectators on Those Parts of the Hospital Containing Women in which he Tactfully Depicts all of the Above-mentioned Types of Madness as They are Found in Them.

Honored Spectators, you have so graciously seen all of the cells, one by one, of those who demonstrate various madnesses and loss of their senses, and who have become a spectacle—more miserable than ridiculous—in the eyes of others,[2] and you have, for the most part, taken as much pleasure in their cases as you could possibly hope for from such novel temperaments, which have provided you, in a single instant—although by different routes—both pleasure and wonderment to your minds with the various types of folly you have seen. Therefore, it now seems to me that it would not be out of the question to show you this other part of the Hospital where women reside and where you can see with your own eyes the most ridiculous examples of feminine madness that you have ever seen in the world. So you will take away from this hospice the greatest pleasure, and you will go through the entire world, filled with great wonderment, telling about and amplifying the horrible follies which I will show you and about which you will learn. And, as you repeat their stories, they will provide the greatest enjoyment to all.

So, I pray you, direct your gaze toward that section which I am pointing out to you, and fix your eyes here, to the left-hand side,[3] where you see that long row of rooms which have so many notes, titles, and emblems above them. These are the cells assigned to madwomen. It is no small privilege to have the opportunity to see them at your ease, since, as a rule, they are rarely shown, and to few people, because of the modesty of their sex, since, as you can see, they are mostly naked.

---

[1] This title has been added for clarity.

[2] Compare 1 Corinthians 4:9–10: "For it seems to me that God has put us apostles on display at the end of the procession, like men condemned to die in the arena. We have been made a spectacle to the whole universe, to angels as well as to men. We are fools for Christ, but you are so wise in Christ! We are weak, but you are strong! You are honored, we are dishonored!"

[3] Aristotle (*Metaphysics*, 5.986a 22–25) attributes right-male left-female dichotomies to the Pythagoreans.

The first chamber which you see with the device hanging over the door depicting a tuft of wild nettles and the motto *In puncto vulnus*, or "A wound in an instant," is the chamber of a Roman matron, Claudia Marcella. In her youth, she was the most sweet, affable, jovial, and delightful girl that you could possibly meet between the two poles. A rare example of loveliness, a unique portrait of courtesy, an image of divine beauty, an expression of the idea of grace and elegance. And now look! What a tragic case hers has been! She slipped with her clogs one day as she was going to the feast of the goddess Buona,[4] and fell on a hard stone, hitting her face and jaw. All of a sudden, losing her senses and her memory, she began to become frenetic and delirious in a way that only became worse. As you see, she sits on her bed, squalid and sick, urinal nearby. Every time you ask her to respond to you about this matter or that, she will take the urinal out of its basket and, looking at herself in it, she says that she is the wise Sibyl, admiring herself, sometimes in the glass, sometimes in the urine. So the Director of our Hospital, an educated and knowledgeable man, has formed that device or emblem on the cause of her sickness, together with that title, wishing to show with dexterity to gentlemen from all over who come to see this part of the Hospital, with that tuft of stinging nettles and by that motto, *In puncto vulnus*, or, "An instant wound," that, like the nettle which, as soon as it touches, immediately stings and torments, so too the matron, as soon as she slipped and fell on the rock, was dealt a cruel blow to her head which was pricked in such a way that she suffers pain and torment in the brutal manner that one sees.

In that other chamber that you see nearby, where you see someone standing in the doorway, silent and sad, eyes turned downward, all disheveled, watching the ground, never lifting her head, but rather with her eyes firmly fixed downward, seemingly absorbed with the ground, is one Martia Cornelia from the region of the Insubrians.[5] She has suffered from melancholic humors since infancy, and that's why you see her so wild in appearance and with such a deathly countenance. And among the other humors that frequently torment her mind, this one is truly cruel: that many times she believes that she has turned into a silkworm, so she does nothing but nibble on mulberry leaves, saying that in this way she is keeping herself alive. Therefore you can readily see that the device and the motto posted over her doorway by the Director correspond to her infirmity. The device is a cocoon with a silkworm inside it and, to one side, a mulberry twig with the motto *Et mihi vitam, et aliis decus*, or "For me, life; for others, beauty."[6]

But please, turn your heads a little way ahead and gaze on that cell with its door open, where the woman has that pincushion and the basket of needles with silk to stitch. But she leaves aside her proper business, and, with that little needle in hand, she goes after flies and spiders instead of doing her embroidery.

---

[4] Buona: Roman goddess of fecundity, also known as the *Bona Dea* or Good Goddess.

[5] "Insubrians": inhabitants of Lombardy.

[6] That is, "the mulberry leaves nourish me and give me life; my silk will provide beautiful clothing for others."

Her name is Marina de' Volsci, so absent-minded and negligent that instead of attending to serious work, she spends the entire day on trifles and whims. So the Director assigned her a device of an old man trying to chase butterflies with the appropriate motto, *Quo gravior eo segnior,* or, "The more serious, the lazier."

The fourth cell, which comes next, if you pay attention—for the door has been thrown wide open—is built in the manner of a tavern. A woman lies prostrate with her hair loose, a thyrsis[7] in her hand, and, nearby, a drum—an instrument to play for the festival of the god Bacchus. She is one of those ancient Maenads, called Bacchae by others, and by still others Stimele, because they are stimulated by the frenzy of Lyaeus. She is called Teronia Elvezia, and with her head full of Greco and Trebbiano wines, she does nothing but whirl around, shaking that thyrsis and beating her drum with all sorts of joyfulness. And finally, really drunk, she stretches herself on the ground in the manner in which you find her now. Because of this, a device was made for her with a motto that reflected her drunkenness. It is none other than a magpie with a mouthful of soup[8] and, under it, these words, *Hinc silens, hinc loquax,* or "Now silent, now talkative."

The next one, whom you see in that cell below, takes up a lantern in order to light her bobbin and spindle even though it is midday and the sun's rays shine on the entire hemisphere. She is a demented and forgetful fool who can remember nothing that she must do. Her name is Orbilia Beneventana.[9] So her device and its motto are very appropriate to her insanity: a mole, which is, by nature, blind, with the motto: *Haec oculis haec mente,* or, "This one, in the eyes; that one, in the mind."[10]

That other truly unhappy and miserable soul, who, as soon as she saw you looking into her cell, hid herself behind that chamber pot and pulled the blanket and the hood over herself, is a certain female called by everyone Lucietta da Sutri. She is so absent in her actions that sometimes, when she goes to light the fire and feels the puff of the bellows, she falls back three yards for fear of that puff. Nor can this sort of thing be removed from her head even though various and sundry physicians have tried a thousand experiments to cure her. Therefore, appropriately, they placed above her door a device showing a rabbit digging in the earth with the motto, *Huic fuga salus,* or "Escape is their salvation,"[11] because, just like a rabbit, she feels safe only when she hides, in the manner that you can see.

---

[7] thyrsis: a giant staff made of fennel and covered with ivy vines and topped with a pine cone. It is a symbol of Bacchus. See above, p. 151, note 15.

[8] A play on "*zuppa*" which means both "soup" as "wine" and "nonsense talk." In Discourse V, *gazze inzuppate* referred to "drunken magpies."

[9] "Orbilia Beneventana" evokes the grammarian Orbilius of Benevento, discussed in Discourse VI. See p. 78, note 6.

[10] In the mole, the eyes are defective; in Orbilia, it is the mind. The emblem echoes Aesop's fable of "The Mole and His Mother," where the mole is not only blind, but also has no sense of smell.

[11] A play on Livy, *nec in fuga salus,* or "nor is there safety in fleeing" (30.8).

If you want to hear a truly demented one, for god's sake, don't miss talking with the next one, all dressed in grey, who has such a gigantic goiter that she could throw it over her shoulder. She is that Menega of Valtolina,[12] daughter of Tognazzo Panada[13] and Matia, his wife, who was once made to believe that a cow had fallen in love with a little frog and, being moved by compassion for her and not knowing any other way of satisfying her, he let her swallow him one day while she was drinking from a river. And then, swimming around inside her, he entered that cavity where the cow conceives. He urinated there and after a term of three years, she gave birth to an animal which had the legs of a frog, with all the rest like a spotted bull like those in Hungary. So, our Director, seeing that she is so round-headed and block-headed,[14] has posted on her cell that device which you see: a buffalo with a ring in its nose and the motto *Quocumque rapior*, or "Lead me anywhere."

In that other cell which you see, there is a certain wretch with as dull and empty a brain as that of any creature in the world that I have seen. Her name is Orsolina Capoana. She has this quality, that if you ask her to sweep the house, she will start to trim her fingernails, and it will be evening before she has completed this task. Sometimes, when she is ordered to prepare the lye for the laundry, she puts her mouth to the spigot of the vat and blows into it—like a madwoman—for three hours. And with similar things, the Miserable One has become so discredited that if you asked her to empty the urinal, you can be sure that, like a little boy with his marbles, or with a thousand other games, she will take at least two hours, and in the end, either she will report back with the box emptied or with the urinal all battered and broken, being the dunce that she is. So don't be surprised if the keeper of the Hospital has placed a device on her door depicting a moth circling a flame with the motto, in Spanish, *Ni mas ni menos*, or, "Neither more nor less," because there is no more stupid creature than a moth, because it circles around until it finally singes its own wings. So there is nothing to compare with the stupidity of this one.

Very similar to her seems this other dull-witted, misguided one. She forgets her spindle while she holds her bobbin next to her. And now, full of amazement, with her eyes staring, she looks toward you as if she had never before seen a man. Her name is Tadia of Pozzuolo, and among her other stupidities is this most notable one: one day, the guard at the Hospital asked her to fetch a little water from the cistern to put on the table. But instead of taking a pail, the idiot took the soup pot in which the cabbage was cooking. She placed that watery broth on the table

---

[12] Valtolina, or Valtellina: a valley in the foothills of the Alps north of Bergamo, already referred to several times, whose inhabitants were known for their stupidity.

[13] "Tognazzo Panada": a name derived from the names of two characters in Folengo's *Baldus:* Barelli, 170, n. 23.

[14] "block-headed," from *grossa di legname*, in Folengo, *Baldus*, 14.51–52: Barelli, 171, n. 24.

in such a way that everyone present was convinced of her melon-headedness, and they shared no little amazement, delight, and amusement. Because of this, she is illustrated with the device which you see: a goose on top of a hedge, with the motto *Frustra nitor*, or, "I struggle in vain."[15] This device with its motto means that just as a goose is more stupid than any other animal, nor can it fly over a hedge, so she does all of the things that she does in a silly manner, because she can do nothing right.

That clumsy simpleton, Margherita of Bologna, seems to be almost of the same brood. She lives in that cell way down at the bottom, and if there were no other signs or vestiges in the world of her clumsiness, this one alone would be more than sufficient: A certain Lady sent her to the pawnshop of the Jews to give him a message from her that she wished to obtain by lease some bracelets and earrings as she usually did for Carnival. She went to the Lady's jewelry chest and took a pair of bracelets which she had in a box, together with some lovely earrings. She brought them to the Jew, saying that the Lady, her mistress, was sending those things to be rented out. She returned from this expedition to her mistress, who was so appalled by this clumsiness that she could not imagine anything worse. Nothing else was talked about in that house for a very long time. So you can see that the custodian has placed an appropriate device over her door: an owl, with the motto *Ipse ego et ego ipse*, or, "It is I, and I am it."

Behold, then, inside the next cell, we come to that wicked Lucilla da Camerino, who is as vicious a fool as possible. To confirm this, just look at the jar that she holds. It is full of walnut extract which turns the skin as black as coal. For hours she has been smearing it all over her body and, naked, goes to accost the ladies of the custodian's household, who have been having their lunch since noon. They are so aghast at such a wretched sight that they all run away, leaving the table as prey to that she-wolf who, without any discretion, does these things to the girls, the maids, and the entire household almost as if they were normal. So above the door to her cell is a device that is appropriate to her: a fox's tail sweeping a room with the French motto, *Par ma foy que liet tan bien*,[16] or "Truly, it cleans equally well."

---

[15] See Erasmus, *Adagia*, "*Frustra niti dementiae est*": 5.2.4. The emblem also evokes Camerarius, *Symbola*, "*Deficiam aut efficiam*," 3.48, "Either I'll reach my goal, or will die trying," also represented by a goose.

[16] Fractured French of obscure meaning. Cherchi suggests substituting "liet" with "niet," obtaining the meaning given in the translation above. The fox's tail is a poor broom, but the fox can "clean up" food from the table extremely well. Similarly, the vicious fool is a poor housekeeper, but is good at cleaning food from the table. Alternatively, Lucilla, like her male counterparts in Discourse XII, excel at repulsing other people, i.e., "sweeping" them away. The motto then reads, "Truly, the fox's tail sweeps out dirt as well as I sweep out people."

I will say nothing to you of that other spiteful fool called Flavia Drusilla whom you see there, together with that puppy. She pets and strokes him so lovingly, as it would seem, but shortly she calls Fiorino to her but he doesn't come, and she flies into such a rage that, out of spite, she would want to strangle him or turn him into jelly. This is her usual way: that for even the smallest thing, she becomes so enflamed with spite that the evil Gabrina or Pinabello's wife[17] would surely lose to her. And if there were nothing else, this event, which happened the other day, is the most serious: while she was doing the laundry, a little lye got into her eye by accident; so this spiteful fool took the laundry tub and threw it against a wall, splintering it. Then she took all of the clothes—which she had washed and then placed in lye—down to a river that runs near here, and threw them all into the stream. Nothing would have been recovered if a good maidservant had not run to the house for help, so they sent servants down with poles to collect them as best they could. So because of this, our Director has had a painter friend of his paint a device over her cell which shows a beaver biting off his own genitals, with the motto *Ulcisci haud melius*, or, "There is no better revenge than this."[18]

Look at that other giraffe in the doorway who does nothing but laugh and smirk, and with every little thing that she sees or hears she throws that mouth wide open like an oven door. Her name is Domicilia Feronia, and she has a husband who shares with her the same stupendous folly. Now because her substance consists of nothing but vulgar laughter, our custodian has placed over her door a little owl[19] on the end of a stick, an animal that would make stones laugh, with the motto, *Haec aliis et mihi alii*, or, "This, others, and others, me."[20] This emblem clearly illustrates her fatuousness which is like a chest full of stuff of all types, but devoid of sense.

I don't know if you can see the one sitting prominently on that seat in her doorway, dressed in that gown which swirls at the bottom not unlike the tail of a peacock. Her name is Tarquinia Venerea, and it is not possible to imagine anyone in the world more vainglorious than she. This will make it clear: One day, as she

---

[17] "Gabrina or Pinabello's wife": two characters from Ariosto's *Orlando Furioso*. For Gabrina, see Discourse XIII, 106–7 n. 8; for Pinabello's wife, see *Orlando Furioso*, 20.110–115 and 22.49–51.

[18] Aelian (*Characteristics of Animals*, 6.34) explains how the beaver castrates himself and by giving the hunters his most valuable parts, saves his own life. The beaver is also mentioned in Pliny, *Natural History*, Aesop, *Fables*, and the emblem books of Alciati, Giovio, and Valeriani in which the self-castrating beaver takes on varied meanings. See Calabritto, "The Subject of Madness," 333–37.

[19] A play on "civetta," which means both "little owl" and "coquette."

[20] In other words, "The owl makes others laugh, and others make me laugh." Aelian (*Characteristics of Animals*, 15.28) explains that there is a little owl which, "if you caricature and imitate them in a playful way [it] affords these birds the greater pleasure. This is the origin of the word *skôptein* which we use, meaning 'to mock'." The motto can then be paraphrased as "I (Domicilia, an owl) make others laugh and others make me laugh."

was telling some gentlemen about her family tree, even though it only goes back less than two hundred years, she said that she was descended from the Queen of Sheba; and she displays a pearl and a diamond of ordinary worth and value which she says the great King Solomon had given to her when she left his court. She insists that everyone believe that these gems had finally been passed down to her. But one day she uttered an even more beautiful story: she told certain ladies who had come to see her that she still kept in her house a pair of taffeta breeches that had belonged to the Lord Consort of her ancestor, the Queen. Therefore, the Director, noting the folly of this simpleton, and fitting a device to her genius, has posted over her cell, as her coat of arms, the image of Time in the manner in which it is depicted by the poets, that is, a snake devouring its own tail, with an appropriate motto, *Sola aeternitate victa*, or, "Defeated only by eternity."[21]

But please, do me this favor, and pay attention to the one who comes next, whose name is Andronica Rodiana. Rest assured that she really is a clever fool because she certainly feigns having lost her mind in order to have a good time. You can tell from this: sometimes she goes to the henhouse and positions herself near the clutch of hens, crying "co co co" to indicate that she has laid an egg. But if you should go to collect the egg, she no longer cries like that, nor preens her feathers or cackles like a hen, but she will pick up a large stick and try to make you stay a long way away from the henhouse. So the Superintendent, noting her behavior, has depicted her as a simulating fool, and has placed above her cell that picture of Fraud with a mis-measuring scale in her hand, and next to it the motto *Ars fortunae salus*, or "The art of fortune is my salvation,"[22] because with these tricks she keeps herself continuously entertained.

Livia of Veletri[23] is the name of that other one whom you see at her window, gazing at the moon, because sometimes one finds her with her senses intact—as if she had never felt the influences of madness—and other times, to the contrary, she shows that she is so stimulated by this passion that, through long experience, they know that she is a lunatic. So the other evening, in her speaking and reasoning, she seemed to be a Minerva; but today, if you ask her something, she cannot keep to the purpose for one second, and she will continuously jump from one topic to another, because as the moon wanes, so does her brain. Therefore, you can see a device with a motto appropriate to this matter: a crab gazing

---

[21] Among the poets, the image of time as a serpent devouring its own tail; an early use of this image (the *ouroboros*) was in Claudian, "On Stilicho's Consulship," 2:428–30 (trans. Platnauer, 2:33). The image was very popular in the Renaissance. The motto also evokes Petrarch, "The Triumph of Time."

[22] The art of manipulating luck or fortune is what saves her.

[23] "Veletri" or "Velletri," a town in the Alban Hills near Rome.

at the shining moon with the motto *Nunc in pleno, nunc in vacuo*, or, "Now full, now empty."[24]

Beautiful Martia Sempronia was committed to the next cell by her relatives. Over the door is painted a winged Cupid with a torch in his hand, with the motto *Desperata salus*, or, "Without hope of rescue."[25] Burning with the flames of love, she went insane a few years ago with love for a certain Quintius Rutilius, and, not knowing what sort of gift she could give to the ungrateful youth in order to lessen his resistance, she cut open a vein with a needle and spilled a copious amount of her blood into a golden cup for him, with a little note attached which said, *Si feris humana prosint*, or "If human things may benefit beasts." This present was found by accident by her brothers and caused her to suffer great tribulation. Therefore, in the midst of reproaches and insults, she became reduced to a desperate degree of amorous madness. She having become completely insane, her family mercilessly confined her to the place that you see.

That woman can be seen to be a companion in a different genus of folly to the next one, who has prepared a noose fastened to that iron hook. Even though her name promises a happy destiny—she is Mansueta[26] Britannia—all of her behaviors are quite to the contrary. Like a desperate fool, she has fastened the noose around her neck three times in order to depart this life, and every time someone has come to her aid. Nor can she be cured of this desperation with remedies of physicians because she has allowed this passion to dominate her too strongly, which is so much less excusable because sometimes she wants to hang herself for trifles. Just the other day she prepared her noose in the manner you see it now, solely because someone had taken one of her sewing needles and she was unable to arrange her pincushion as she had wanted to. Therefore her device and motto reflect her extreme desperation: the device is the trunk of a cypress tree[27] which, when once cut, will never grow again, and the motto is *Semel mortua quiescam*, or, "Once dead, I shall rest."

---

[24] According to the astrologers, the crab, representing the constellation Cancer, is ruled by the waxing and waning of the moon which was thought to be in the constellation Cancer at the time that the world was formed. Garzoni may here be mocking astrology in keeping with post-Tridentine dictates. See Camerarius, *Symbola "Ad Motum Lunae,"* 4.51: "Bring the moon close, and I take it too; move it away and I will also weaken; can the image of hope be any better illustrated?" See also Aelian, *Characteristics of Animals*, 9.6: " . . . as the moon moves [crabs] are in the habit of somehow becoming both emptier and lighter."

[25] In classic Greek society, the bride would be accompanied to the marriage bed by torches. Martia's emblem evokes the story of Dido's desperate love of Aeneas, her preparation of her own funeral pyre, and her suicide by stabbing: Virgil, *Aeneid*, 4.

[26] "Mansueta," meaning "docile."

[27] In Alciati's *Emblemata* (number 199) the cypress tree is a symbol of death. Twigs of cypress were used as funeral decorations. The tree was thought not to bear fruit, hence its association with death.

Who would not say that Ortensia Quintilia—the one lives in the cell at the bottom—is a sister of Ortensio of Bergamo or of Sarni,[28] since she is a slick fool just like him? Because if her stuff is not shown to be the same as his, they can both go and hang themselves. To show you the truth of what I have said, she is so lacking in intellect and her brain is so crippled that one day, as she sat next to the fire idly poking at a burning log with tongs, she took delight in watching the many sparks fly up, which children call nickels and dimes to their fathers' amusement.[29] But the maid was skimming the pot and splashed enough broth onto the logs that she extinguished the fool's enjoyment and brought great difficulties onto herself, because the infuriated madwoman picked up the burning log by one end and ran after the servant throughout the neighborhood, crying, "After him! After that lazybones!" Suffice it to say that the matter became known by the maid's own report and by others in the household, and, growing worse day by day, as happens in these cases, she was forced by her family to let them take her here where the guardian of the Hospital, fully informed of her humors, composed the device which you see, and placed it above her cell. It is nothing else but a green pear struck by a large hailstone, with the motto *Actum est*,[30] or, "It is ripe," which wonderfully accords with her folly which is certainly absolutely hopeless.

Now cheer up a little and lift your spirits by observing that clown, Terenzia the Samnite, who in her gestures, her words, her bearing, and her stories seems to be Boccafresca's sister or Gonella's daughter.[31] As an indication of this, the other day she sat down at a desk, and called together in her room nearly the entire family of the Director. They all hurried to hear some wonderful idea, as usual, from her. Many people made a circle around her, expecting some discourse or sermon as she commonly gave at other times. But this time—and not without laughter—she made a thousand gestures with her hands and eyes, first this way, then that, always seeming to want to be about to begin right then. Finally, she produced a gigantic belch like a hog, and said that she had not assembled them for any other reason but that such a noble belch should be honored by a large assembly such as this. Therefore, that device that you see above her cell is most appropriate to her: a head of

---

[28] "Ortensio of Bergamo or Sarni": possibly a reference to the "Ortensio of Sarni" of Discourse X. See Fiorato, n. 813.

[29] A reference to the Italian superstition that one can foretell the future by noting the way sparks fly off of the burning logs. Children would count the sparks and demand coins from their fathers based on their count: Cherchi, 366, n. 56.

[30] This adage can be found in Erasmus, *Adagia*, 1.3.39 (31: 268–69).

[31] "Boccafresca . . . Gonella." We met Boccafresca and Gonella in Discourse XXI, where they are described as clowns or buffoons. See 147nn. 22–23 above.

Zani[32] with German breeches at his nose, with the motto in Germanized Italian,[33] *Chesta stare buone compagne,* or "This is good, friends."

Quintia Emilia has a most sweet temperament, pleasant and jovial, born for the pleasure and amusement of everyone. She occupies the lowest cell, and has three gentlemen with her to whom she gives wonderful entertainment with her speech. Not long ago, one of them asked her when women are most foolish, and she wittily replied, "When you men allow them room to be foolish." Another asked her "Why has nature given women such small brains?" She cleverly responded that, given the truth of his statement, the reason was obvious: Nature acted like the female that she is. So it is enough that there is an appropriate device for her which depicts Jupiter on a golden throne in the center of the heavens with the motto from the poet, *Iovis omnia plena,*[34] or, "All things are full of Jupiter."

Look at that bizarre and capricious Erminia of Bohemia who put the entire household into an uproar the other day over a roasted chestnut, and now she gives them to everybody, whether they want them or not. The other day she cried with her neighbor, Marietta, for more than an hour over a dried apple, and then made peace in an instant. She merits the device that hangs above her cell: an Indian rooster that ruffles its feathers in an instant and then, immediately stops, with the motto *Tanto lenis quanto propera,* or, "Gentle as you are, so hasten."

The woman who is chained to her bed nearby is a real bestial fool called Giacoma of Piangipane,[35] who played this lovely prank the other day: a lad came up to her to empty her chamber pot and she picked it up and mercilessly hit him on the head with it, so that it was three days before the poor boy was himself again. The day before yesterday, she played another one that was even more polished. She came upon a donkey that had by chance entered this place with two boxes full of eggs on its back. She picked up a rake used to rake up the grain, and so persecuted him that she made him fall into that ditch which serves as a drain for this place's sewage. The poor beast got stuck with his entire load and broke all of the eggs in the box. Next, she assaulted the donkey's master, who was walking behind him, and if he had not quickly pulled back, I have no doubt whatsoever that she would have beaten his head into a giant frittata. Therefore, our Director, mindful of this fool's bestial temperament, has had depicted above her cell a disheveled Megaera[36] with the motto, *Accensa nil dirius,* or "Nothing more ferocious than one set aflame."

A short way down, take a good look at that one who stands pensively, looking toward the wall, with her thoughts totally fixed on it. She is Lavinia the Ae-

---

[32] "Zani": nickname for Giovanni, one of the most famous of the masks of the Commedia dell'Arte, from which we get "zany." .

[33] There is no German in this motto: it is fractured or macaronic Italian.

[34] Virgil, *Bucolics,* 2.60. Also compare Erasmus, *Adagia, Jovis et regis cerebrum,* 1.6.60.

[35] Piangipane: a town west of Ravenna.

[36] One of the Furies or Erinyes.

tolian, who is an extravagant and witless fool. I know because of this: not long ago she wrote a note to an important princess at an address similar to the one used by those people in San Marino in Romagna when they wrote to the Council of Venice. She said, "To our dear and beloved sister, the Republic of Venice," because those people of San Marino, even though they are almost all peasants, live in a republic just like the Venetian Councillors. In that note, she asked them a favor: that she would come to visit them with all of her maids, and stay with her for eight days, and she would put in order a palace fit for a Cleopatra. Among other delights, she would give a gift of a beaver's testicle[37]—not like the one that a friend of mine from Piacenza bought from a rascal in the city of Trevigi, but a little smaller—which would serve to perfume the cabbage soup, it was so special and precious. And to each of her damsels, she would give a present of an Indian cricket which awakens people without a clock at whatever time they wish. Therefore, above this fantastic being, the device that you see has been created: the image of the monstrous Medusa with the motto *Extrema peto* or "I strive for the extreme," because it is certain that her temperament is nothing if it is not monstrous and extreme.[38]

Following right after her is a fool who, for all of her activities, gets nothing but blows. Her name is Calidonia da Eppi. She never stops, and never calms down, first mocking this one, then sneering at that one, then, grabbing her key, she returns home either with her face all scratched up or with her hair in a mess, or her mouth busted, because these are the desserts which usually come to her after meals. So her device is a plucked hen with the motto *Quid nostra prosunt*? or, "What good are our things?" One knows immediately in what way she errs.

The one further on, called Cecilia Venusia, is a reckless fool who is constantly involved in buffoonery. Nor can one find a prettier coquette than she, so that she always has a coterie of women around her who would certainly be dead or lost without her. With her buffoonery, her various nonsense rhymes and satires, with her telling a thousand tales, more wonderful than those of Straparola,[39] with her chattering more than a parrot, she has introduced here such delightful times that all melancholic and unruly humors are swept away. So, because of this, you can well understand why her *impresa* is a crown for a tavern on the tip of a stick,[40]

---

[37] See p. 194 n. 18.

[38] The motto recalls *summa petit* ("it aspires to [or strives after] the highest things") in Bargagli's collection (*La prima parte dell'imprese* [Siena: Bonetti, 1578]) where they accompany the image of fire going upward and refer to Livy's description of Envy.

[39] Straparola: Giovanni Francesco Straparola (1495–1557), author of a popular collection of stories, *The Pleasant Nights (Le piacevoli notti*, 1552), Fiorato notes that Straparola is the only writer mentioned by Garzoni who was known for his "modern" stories and anecdotes: Fiorato, n. 841.

[40] A typical sign of a tavern at the time. See Fiorato, n. 842.

with the motto *Undique risus*, or, "Laughter everywhere," because this device and motto could not fit anyone better than her.

Next comes Armolia Filisca, an Unbridled Fool, like a horse. She is licentious in all of her activities and out of control with all of her words, and, with reckless freedom, she rants and raves at everyone. Just the other day, seeing a large crowd of gentlewomen coming from a celebration, she finally said that a hairpin was not positioned appropriately on the cloth around the head of one of them as it should be. Therefore her device is a horse's bridle with the motto *Nil satius*, or, "Nothing is enough," since she is very well known for being that fearless madwoman, which is what she truly is.

The next-to-last cell belongs to Laurentia Giglia, an Obstinate Fool, like a mule, in all of her doings. One can clearly appreciate her obstinacy by this: a few days ago, having been screamed at by her family for standing at her window and talking with I-don't-know-who, she immediately left, and then returned again. When they screamed at her again, she withdrew inside and then reappeared. Neither the wind nor a great rainstorm mixed with hailstones bigger than eggs could budge her from that spot, since she was determined to win the battle against heaven and earth. Therefore, with good reason, they have assigned her a device showing an anvil being struck by a hammer, with the motto *Nec ictibus scissa*, or, "Unbroken even by blows," which clearly signifies the extreme obstinacy that she has in her head.

But the one who completes our rabble, who finishes off our revelry, and who prepares the party as it should be, is Ostilia from Modena, either Merlin's sister or Calcabrino's daughter,[41] an inspired woman, diabolical, and full of all sorts of wickedness. This devilish fool is so monstrous and malignant that there is no device in the world that can adequately signify her perverse, iniquitous, and abominable nature. Therefore she alone, among all the others, is left without an *impresa* or any image. Neither Gabrina for spite, nor Circe for diabolical enchantments, nor any other monster celebrated by the ancients could aptly represent her monstrous and tremendous properties. And therefore, honorable spectators, I conclude that it would be better for you not to approach her cell for any reason, because if she becomes aware of your presence here, be assured that, like an Alcina, she will transform you all into beasts or into plants or stones. And as a reward for entering into a Hospital of Fools, you will find yourself in that palace where the wicked enchantress transforms men into donkeys. This is what you might get from her.

So let us close the gates of the Hospital, and leave. Keep your distance, for you have seen more than enough.

---

[41] "Calcabrino": the enraged demon who pursues Dante (*Inferno* 22 and 23). In Discourse XXX, on diabolical madmen, she is called "Calubrino" (183).

Poems[1] by Teodoro Angelucci[2] to Tomaso Garzoni:
On Madness

Last night, in my cloak, when I read
Your *Hospital*, my dearest Garzoni,
I felt my head spinning
Because that God who presides over buffoons,
And carries a lantern to the other stars,
Lifted his thigh above his balls,
Relaxed the hole from his internal valley
And warmed up my brain, that was frozen,
With his fraternal wind;
So I returned home all upset
And, without greeting the maid,
I took pen in hand, as if insane.
For now my beloved muse
Does not mess with arms and lovers,[3]
As if she scorned lofty subjects.
She prepares to sing of madness
Against which swords and stronger
Virtues are impotent;
But why am I holding you up
And not beginning my song,
Telling of the frenzy that now delights me?
When the first rays of sunlight shone forth
And festive Nature revealed

---

[1] These poems were originally in *terza rima*, the classical form employed by Dante and many other classical Italian poets. Garzoni's intent was to give these poems on madness a lofty, classical feel. We offer here a free verse rendition of these poems.

[2] Teodoro Angelucci, born in Belforte, physician and philosopher; wrote a dedicatory poem for Garzoni's *Piazza*. See also the Introduction, p. 3ff and notes.

[3] "arms and lovers": echos the first line of *Orlando Furioso*, "Of ladies, cavaliers, of love and war," itself playing off of Vergil's *Arma virumque*.

Her never-seen shoulders,
Lovely things were scattered and freely roamed
Here and there throughout the world,
And goodness was divided into many parts;
Until, thanks to a benign star,
They all joined together
To form a much more beautiful thing.
Therefore madness is not of just one seed
But splits up into many branches,
And is still found in the most distant twigs.
Let the wise man wish for
The sameness all the time, and always
Reduce to reason both the place and the meaning;
As you well know, O Garzoni, this habit is born from having
Little or nothing in one's head, for where
There is a paucity of firewood, there too the fire is weak.
Each man looks up to High Jupiter
As to the sovereign and eternal good
Because he breaks up into several new graces;
A sophist may say that it is not appropriate
To argue this, because great evil and no good
Ever comes from the temperament of madness;
Now wrath really rises up to the tip of my nose
And I would crush such a man
Like an eggshell were he to stand before me;
For I do not find, by nature,
That what is desired by most
Is most often some evil, old or new.
But all things incline toward the beloved good,
And for the most part they also choose goodness
If they are not kept from doing so by force.
What god could restrain the fast and precipitous
Race of innumerable people towards madness,
With certain fear or with assured hope?
Therefore according to philosophy
To have a foolish brain is a good thing;
And to be wise is something trite and wrong:
Haven't poets, musicians, and painters held
High esteem and the garland above all else?
And where does the name *literati* not resound?
Aren't soldiers much better perhaps
Than those who idly spend their time sweetly
Lying belly-down among grasses and flowers?

And yet these are all clearly
More foolish and capricious than other men;
Even if they wrongly say it is otherwise,
Now among illusions, now among sorrowful thoughts,
Now in the air of vain and false honor,
Now among the hidden secrets of nature,
They afflict their souls so much that the final fruits
Of their errors are the chains:
That great remedy which can tame any humor.
I recall that Bellerophon [4]
Who ended up living a solitary life in the woods;
Ajax, who slashed his own veins; [5]
Hercules, who ended his own life
In flames; [6] Empedocles and Plato, [7]
Who wrote so well and learnedly;
And many most serious persons
Who gave the ultimate boot to reason
Precisely because they were so illustrious.
Vile or crude is the heart that does not feel
The wicked torments of love, and it is also great folly
For two eyes to die chaste and happy.
What more accursed trap is there
Than that which, if anyone puts his foot into it,
Traps his sweet freedom forever?
Whoever saw a man who believes he is wise
Go around naked during the summer
When the angry dog beats down on the earth? [8]
Madmen, in every place and age,
Are allowed to satisfy any wish

---

[4] Bellerophon was sent by Proteus with a letter to Iobates in which the latter was requested to put him to death. At Iobates' request he killed the Chimaera. Homer (*Iliad*, 6. 155–202), reports that "when Bellerophon came to be hated by all the gods, he wandered all desolate and dismayed upon the Alean plain, gnawing at his own heart, and shunning the path of man" (trans. Samuel Butler). See Brumble, *Myths*, 54–56.

[5] Ajax contended with Ulysses for the possession of Achilles' weapons. When they were assigned to Ulysses he became insane and killed himself. Cf. p. 157, note 2.

[6] Hercules leapt into the flames of Mt. Oeta. Cf. p. 157, note 1.

[7] Empedocles and Plato: Empedocles' madness is dealt with in Discourse XV. Plato's "madness" goes back to the notion of the poet's *furor*.

[8] "angry dog": The ancients believed that when Sirius, the brightest star in the constellation Canis Major, was in conjunction with the sun, its heat, together with that of the sun, was responsible for the summer heat—"the dog days of summer."

As if they were blessed souls;
Some wise men tried to teach
A less boring life to miserable mortal men
In order to acquire glorious fame for themselves,
Imitating madmen and animals
Who follow simple nature.
To tell good from evil,
They would eat and sleep at random;
They relieved their bodies, and planted their manhood
Wherever they pleased, without fear:
Quietly, they would spin in all directions in their barrels:[9]
In the air, in shade, and in sunlight,
And sowed silver and gold in the sea.
But since, in fact, in order to function well,
It is necessary to do everything according to nature,
Not with falsity and with words,
These men lived too wisely,
And did not have a happy life
Like those who are completely crazy.
I speak so, because, whether a little or a lot,
Everyone participates in the beginnings of madness,
As that poet says.[10]
So I conclude, that to live loosely,
And like a real madman, is more natural to man
Than to have his spirit convoluted by many rules;
What safety then may equal
Madness if, to be mad
Is the only good defense for any offense?
No one believes it is a fair or honest act
To avenge a slap or blow
Inflicted by a madman, or when he contends for someone's path.
And madmen live the fullest and most
Lives, because they cleverly
Mix up both false and true things.
And if I well penetrate into this with my reason,
They are certainly right, since they imitate God,
To whom the first honors are everywhere given.

---

[9] An allusion to Diogenes of Sinope (412–323 B.C.) who is said to have lived in a barrel. He despised the lofty musings of "wise men," and when Alexander the Great asked him what he could do for him, he said, "Get out of the sunlight." His followers were the Cynics, whose behavior is described here.

[10] "the poet": Ariosto, *Orlando Furioso*, especially Canto 34, 85.

He has the characteristic of deriving good
From both good and evil,
And evil or bad men never came from him.
Therefore a madman—while he keeps as his own
The property of others, and has the membranes
Of his brain filled with false and imaginary ghosts—
Is like a man who drank salt water
Instead of fresh, in his extreme thirst,
And thereby rendered his lungs humid and cold.
But further, I say to you, who are learned men,
And who diligently peruse ancient parchments:
That beacon, more eternal than the world,
And which people call Truth,
Governs the crazy more than it does the wise.
And the thing they call Honesty,
That great queen of prudent men,
From whom all virtues are born,
Is nothing but a fine illusion
Of vain and idle poets.
Man cultivates it in order to lose himself.
For this reason, men of letters were noxious
To the large crowd of evil people
As if they were rebellious and unruly.
Do you, Garzoni, wish to understand this? Then listen,
While I sing four more lines,
And may your mind be focused on me alone.
Each one imagines and adorns this Prudence
As he likes: some remove afflictions
From the honest man; others strain
To moderate their foul passions,
So that they may become wise; and what one says
Makes souls servants to high virtue,
Another—clever and untimely—insists
That it is something vicious. The two never cease arguing,
Until someone takes them out.
They all agree in surrounding their virtues
With pungent thorns, and describe them as being
Close to impossible.
I never saw or read that, among mortals,
(I speak according to nature) no more than one or two
Were really virtuous
The way they want an honest man
And one who is called wise to be

A just touchstone for others and for himself.
Therefore it is a fable and the empty words
Of our wise men, to say that virtue can be found
Without madness in mortal man.
So one can always find that the true cause
Of a madman's behavior is some kind of folly;
Whether from the usual humors or new ones.
But whoever thinks he has found
The real and manifest reason for wise acts
Is a great simpleton in the judgment of the learned.
The reason is this: smoke,
Air, illusions, and wind adhere with
Difficulty to our brains.
In many places, I saw hundreds
Of wise men go irrevocably mad
In an instant, in a moment;
But those who are accustomed to folly
Will not grow wise in fifty years,
Unless they are prodded with a stick.
Therefore, Garzoni, agree with me this instant:
Folly is natural to us,
And wisdom is an unbearable torment.
Water that has been heated for many hours, once
It is removed from the fire, soon and quickly
Returns jubilantly to its coldness,
Because the scalding heat, according to the universal
Judgment of the learned, is noxious to it
And contrary by nature.
Can't you see that no wise man is worth
Keeping your laughter in your pocket for,
Nor for the fun of seeing a great fool? Or how everybody
Is flooded with embarrassment, and bitterness
Distorts one's features when he looks at
Someone that he esteems to be a wise man?
Not only do men willingly tend
To madness, but the vain gods, too,
Love anybody whose brain spins.
So, in the old days, the demigods
Were loaded up and full of divine frenzy.
Yet I would call that frenzy madness.
The priests who—day and night—

Served Apollo, Dindymene,[11]
Or Dionysus as their destinies
Were not all, as everyone well knows,
Completely devoid of reason;
And were their gestures and voices not full of fury?
I add—although you are shy with people—
That Mohammed taught the Turks
To honor madmen both dead and alive.
But perhaps these are fables. I know that I read
In holy writ that Holy Ghosts
Are crazy to our mortal intellect.
If you ask me to place before you
All sorts and types of folly,
Listen a little longer to my short song.
Everybody should easily be convinced
That for each of the many planets as there are in the sky,
There is an equal number of types of madness—
Whether fresh or inborn.
Our mortal globe
Is moved by the eternal celestial sky,
And is governed by it down to a hair's-breadth.
Saturnines are like soups,
Whether cold or reheated: they are tasteless.
When one greets them from the window,
They are quite harsh in their gestures and in their talk.
They wear large, wide hats,
And other than while practicing usury, they are always cold.
Jovials give their own stuff to their friends
Without need of a whip or spurs.
They are light in offenses, and easy to forgive.
They so hate weeping and complaints
That about death itself they promptly laugh.
It's not a bad thing that their joy lingers on.
Martials live on human blood.
They eat dead-bolts and armored vests.
In cursing, if they are doing well, they shriek.
They shoot with artillery; they spit out the spoils
Of men by the thousands, and when they speak

---

[11] "Dindymene" is Cybele or Rhea, the goddess who was worshipped on Mount Dindymus or Dindymon. She was worshipped by the Corybantes, her enthusiastic priests who, with drums, cymbals, horns, and full armor, performed orgiastic dances in the forests and mountaintops of Phrygia. See Brumble, *Myths*, 85–87, 77–79.

The neighboring towns tremble.
Then the sunny madmen[12] burst
With blind ambition, and they walk all day
Just to have two greetings with the hat.
If by chance they are the last to sit,
They develop an acute fever in their hearts for the next three months
And are delirious for entire days and nights.
Each tongue would be dry and dumb[13]
While telling of your madmen, beautiful Venus,
Born in the sea, amid pearls and corals.
A lover, in order to hear news
From his dearly beloved goddess
Through the words of a lying old woman,
Does not avoid perils, nor expense,
Does not feel the heat or the ice, or the other evils
Of the cold or of the summer season.
In his mouth he always has the loving darts,
The torches, the arrows, the curly hair,
Amaranthine reds, lily whites, and things like that.[14]
The strolls, the sighs, the humble bows,
The weeping, the gazes, the hand-kissings,
The little shoes, the strands of hair, the feathers
Are not above the indicators of these vain ones.
But to despair and to bang one's head on the wall
Are things, by my faith, that are worthy of men who are more than mad.
Mercury's madmen were always
Different: pimps, gossips,
And thieves that have a secret name.
To these then we must add the buffoons,
The learned, the curious, the charlatans,
The smoky alchemists, and the spies.
But where have I left those strange fools
Of the inconstant so-called tri-form goddess[15]
Who are often far from themselves?
The unstable lunatic running

---

[12] "sunny madmen": Apollonians.

[13] The line echoes Dante: "… ch' ogne lingua deven tremando muta" ("… that each tongue, quivering, became mute"): *Vita nuova*, 26.1. 3.

[14] "Amaranthine reds, lily whites": the colors of the beloved's lips and skin.

[15] "tri-form goddess": Luna or Semele, goddess of the moon.

From thought to thought until he falls asleep[16]
Is like naked, formless matter;
Now he holds something dear and now he abhors it
And when you try to make a deal with him
You can never get a straight answer.
But my leisure for singing has already ended.
It is now time to get back to the question.
Therefore, peace be with you,
See you again, away from madness.

---

[16] "thought to thought" echos Petrarch, *Canzoniere*, 129, v. 1. "From thought to thought, mountain to mountain top / Love leads me on . . . " (trans. Musa). See also the Introduction, p. 3 and note.

Poem
In Praise of Madness
by Signor Guido Casoni[1]

Muses, I greet you until the day I see you again.
I have just now departed with my dear Signor Frenzy
To spend a short time with madness,
To discover his virtues, which have been neglected
By those who praised syphilis, the needle, the spindle,
The ass, the fig, and the radish.[2]
And this holy sir, whom it is customary nowadays
To neglect, is such a universally noble man,
Useful and necessary to human life!
If man laments that he is mortal
He can also boast that he is mad.
O sweet comfort for such evil:
You, sweet and pious nourisher of thoughts,
Veritable sun who casts away pain from the mind,
Opposite of evil, holy madness.
While in the sweet shade of your banner
I write about you—for you—I pray that you lend me
Rhymes, and fill my brain with lofty concepts;
For if you minister to my words,
Rest assured that Burchiello, Bernia, and Tansillo[3]
Will be revered by me and will stand to my left.

---

[1] Guido Casoni, born in Serravalle (modern Vittorio Veneto) in 1561; died 1542. Lawyer and poet. Was a member of the Accademia dei Perseveranti and the Accademia degli Incogniti and wrote a biography of Tasso. Some of his poetry is collected in *Opere scelte di Giovan Battista Marino e dei Marinisti*, ed. G. Getto (Turin: Utet, 1954). Barelli, 198, n. 1. See also the Introduction, p. 2 and note 5.

[2] "syphilis . . . radish": objects praised by various authors, e.g., syphilis by Bini, the needle by Berni, the spindle by G. Ruscelli, the fig by Francesco Maria Molza: Barelli, 198, n. 2.

[3] "Burchiello, Bernia, and Tansillo": the first two were mentioned by Garzoni in Discourse XXVIII, where they are considered among the "madmen frenetic, like a

But while I sail the tranquil seas
Of your praise, and I empty out—drop by drop—
That capacious vessel with the small opening,[4]
Prepare the laurel. Not the one of Parnassus,
But the one for eels, that may emit an odor
That would make Gnatho rush to follow his nose.[5]
Well, now, I'll start. If your great favor
Makes one's brain spin, even the sky, which constantly
Spins, pays tribute and honor to you.
In fact, lady Dawn appears first,
Crowned with flowers, then fierce golden Phoebus,
And then the sky puts out its beautiful mantle
So that the globe on which we live,
Being adorned with so many different and gentle things,
Makes men fall in love with it.
Nor does it look like Nature completely scorns
Your lofty qualities. In fact we see that she
Often immerses herself in your sweetness.
She enjoys making one woman adorned and beautiful,
And another one with a distorted and odd appearance;
One courteous and another foul and rebellious.
She relishes making a healthy person a poor slave,
And a rich one sickly; and placing a wise man in a lowly position
While placing the scepter in the hands of a reckless man.
In smiling May, she enjoys promising
To enrich the soil with a thousand favors,
To shower milk, and make the beech tree drip honey.
And then she pesters hay, grapes, grass, and flowers
With hail, and rips them up with the wind,
Taking back her favors like an ungrateful woman.
And we, considering the events alone,
Do not know that these accidents
Fall upon us for an ultimate good end.
But I would completely fill this page
If I tried to explain
How everything contains madness.
Then you would think that I had nothing
To say about its royal place

---

horse." They were satirical, non-conformist writers of the sixteenth century who all had difficulties with church authoritites because of their anti-establishment writings.

[4] That capacious vessel: *Orlando Furioso*, 23.113.

[5] Gnatho: proverbial parasite and sycophant of Terence's *Eunuch*.

And that I had passed over in silence what imports most.
If Madness were to die without an heir,
It has been established by the legislators
That man should, by rights, succeed it.
Here I see you stop and say, with a smile,
If man and Madness are related,
How can one be separated from the other?
I reply, that the legislators
Were contemplative philosophers, and in each doubtful instance
They gave their opinion without being influenced by feelings.
More than once they had read
That each worldly thing inclines towards its end.
So they inferred that man must be the heir to folly.
The reason is, that an inheritance goes
To the next-of-kin.
And no one else competes for being more closely related.
Venus in the heavens
Is not so clear and resplendent
As she is when she shines on the heads of mortals—
The more intensely, the more worthy is the man.
Some are more, some are less; people are not all the same,
But they are all crazy,[6]
And let's leave aside the other animals for now.
They all receive the venerable gift,
Some in dancing, some in fencing with a sword,
Some in singing, and some in playing music,
Some in filling streets with majesty
By wearing stripe-bedecked caps and feathers,
And by distilling manna and dew from their noses;
Some in serving an angelical, divine
Face, and then, weeping, calling the heavens
Cruel, and evil, and their destiny unfair;
Some in honors, some in making money,
Some in being taken up with hopes of a lord's favors
Which are sterile or rarely delivered;
Some in sailing the sea; some in seeing
Many lands; some in seeking gold beneath the ground;
Some in being courteous courtiers;
Some in seeking news of the wars

---

[6] Here begins a section that recalls again *Orlando Furioso*, 34.85.

In Persia and in Flanders,[7] and what is happening in Rome
And the rest of the world;
Some in browsing the ancient histories and the new ones
With Berossus, Herodotus, and Tarcagnota;[8]
Some in seeing what persuades and moves;
Some in seeking to acquire
The power of argumentation; some in discovering
Everything about point, line, and surface;
Others in putting every effort into learning
The most hidden secrets of Nature;
Others in forever building astrolabes and spheres;
Some in putting all of their attention into learning
Arithmetic, the law, and medicine,
The cabala, and the dark Raimondina.[9]
But above all the arts and sciences, the ones inclining towards
Madness the most are alchemy, painting,
And having the divine grace of poetry.
O revered honor above all others!
O happy Melitidis and Coroebus,[10]
So famous for such great favor.
Ulysses knew that madmen are blessed,
So he feigned madness;[11] and strong Orlando,[12]
Cleomedes,[13] and Hercules[14] were celebrated as such.
Her lofty dignity was known when
Mother Nature placed her in the brain,
Recognizing she was worthy of governance.

---

[7] Persia and Flanders: sites of the wars over the Holy Land and the insurrections countered by Philip II, respectively.

[8] Three historians who all have in common important works on Babylon. See *The Babyloniaca of Berossus*, ed. Stanley Burstein (Malibu: Undina Publications, 1978); Giovanni Tarcagnota, *Delle historie del mondo* (Venice: Vorischi, 1617).

[9] "Raimondina": a reference to the mystical, occult writings of Raymon Lull. See also p. 51, note 46.

[10] Melitidis: the proverbial fool of Erasmus's "*Melitidis auxilium*," or "The assistance of Melitidis." He is included in Discourse XI, "Clumsy and Fatuous Fools." "Coroebus" is another object of an Erasmus adage, "*Stultior Coroebo*," or "More foolish than Coroebus." See Discourse VI, "Forgetful and Demented Madmen," See also p. 97, note 2 and p. 78, note 10.

[11] Ulysses: regarding his feigning madness, see Discourse XVI.

[12] Orlando: the frenzied hero of Ariosto's epic *Orlando Furioso* as well as other popular romances of the time.

[13] Cleomedes: discussed in Discourse XIII.

[14] Hercules: discussed in Discourses XVIII, XXV, and XXVIII.

And she placed her above the servile limbs,
So that she would be a teacher and a guide for their operations;
And deservedly, she gave her preeminence,
Because she leads man to the real good,
For, in a madman, illustrious ancestors, gold,
Power, or beauty induce no pride.
He does not care to possess gems or treasures,
Nor does he strain to please the senses;
Nor does he give rest to his sweat with idleness.
He does not let his heart become prey to intense hatred;
And it never happens that, like a new Philoxenus,[15]
He thinks of abundant food and exquisite wine.
He is not full of envy like Zoilus[16] or like Asinius,[17]
But, content and merry, he always rests
In the arms of tranquil peace.
Therefore, holy Madness, who so likes
To do good, and by means of which the world
Is full of so much glory, and lives in peace,
Oh, why can't I enjoy your favor, so fecund,
So that I may elevate you to such a lofty position
That you could see that, through you, everybody is happy?
I have no shortage of praise while I am praising you,
It's just that time is short as I write;
The table is set, and I hear them calling me.
But I will quickly describe a case to you,
Where you will see the value of madness,
And so that I may speedily get this over with.
A nobleman there is, whose stars were so benign
At birth that all his desires are satisfied,
And he harvests every sweetness of this life.

---

[15] Philoxenus (fl. ca. 400 B.C.): Athenaeus reports on the authority of Clearchus that Philoxenus would roam the city with his slaves carrying oil, wine, fish-paste, vinegar, and other relishes and would enter a house, unannounced, and begin to season the food to his liking. Athenaeus has many anecdotes about him (*Deipnosophists*, 1.25). Also in Tixier, *Officina*, 7.

[16] Zoilus (400-320 B.C.): Greek rhetorician and philosopher, he was a proverbial carping critic. He chastised Homer for telling fables; hence, a generally critical or censorius person. In Tixier, *Officina*, 7, and Manuzio, *Adagia* (859).

[17] Asinius: Gaius Asinius Pollio (75 or 76 B.C.-5 A.D.) was of fiery ambition. At the age of 22, he came forward as the accuser of C. Cato. He was known for his severe judgment of his contemporaries. He pointed out many mistakes in Cicero and faulted Sallust for his antiquated language. In Tixier, *Officina*, 7.

Thanks to madness, he has not only silver,
Gold, villas, cities, provinces and kingdoms,
But the entire universe is at his disposal.
And being in power, he creates great projects:
Drying out the seas and lowering great mountains,
So that he may make an eternal mark.
It seems to him that everybody is ready
To obey him; he distributes honors;
He ordains kings, generals, marquises, and counts.
There is no region of the world so far away
That it does not pay tribute to him; and now he receives
The Japanese, at great expense and planning,
Six thousand servants chosen for his service,
And six thousand maids. As for the rest
Of the court, you can judge for yourselves.
Isn't this a happy, merry life?
O dear, sweet, blessed Madness
Through which so much good is made manifest to us!
The end is here; I suggest you hurry.

To Angelucci: In Praise of Madness by the Author

My dear Angelucci, a certain whim,
Or perhaps a humor, or a bizarre mood—
Worse than the one that Master Grillo had[1]—
Is constantly troubling my mind,
So I can—continuing in a slapdash manner—
Sing with you of the qualitites of Madness.
But I don't know if I will write something good
Because I have fallen into disfavor with the Muses,
And I was cheated by them like a monkey.
By God, I have, enclosed within my brain,
So much material on this topic
That I would purr to Bernia and Burchiello.[2]
But the Muses, seeing that I want to use them
For my concept, have plotted together
To scorn me as much as they can.
I see that my hope of their favor is gone,
So that only the whim is left for me
To show that I have some kernel of poetry.
But if I follow my brain in flight,
Like those who gave form to Buovo and Ancroia,[3]
(You know that I have just rented the lyre)
Please excuse me, you who are the joy
Of the Aonian[4] chorus, and you who have grown weary
Of *Morgante* and similar writings.

---

[1] "Maestro Grillo," or "Master of the Grasshoppers": See p. 43, note 16.

[2] See p. 175, note 11 and p. 211, note 3.

[3] Buovo and Anacroia: heroes of popular romances of the time. Buovo or Buovio was the hero of the Charlemagne romance "Bevis of Hamton." In Luigi Pulci's *The Epic Adventures of Orlando and His Giant Friend Morgante*, Buovo is Orlando's uncle.

[4] In Aonia, in Boeotia, is Mount Helicon and the fountain Aganippe, sacred to the Muses.

Not everyone can sing with a golden plectrum.
I am content if, with the sound of my theorbo,[5] I can
Awake some of them.
And if people are not moved by such a sound,
What am I to do? I think I need
To get the clapper of the big bell,[6]
And with the help of Pedrala and Togna,[7]
Playing Merlin among the brigade,[8]
With a pumpkin at least scratch the itch,
So that I may not create a disaster in the end.
I will at least try to fit my clumsy argument to my tune
With Gradella on the stage.[9]
And if I seem to some a mountebank,
My excuse will be the topic that I chose,
In itself deserving of no less.
Come on now, since the circle has now formed,
Come forward, and may the whole world hear,
Whether I well spent my five coins in singing.
From the beginning I want to take off my gloves
And begin such a serious praise that,
In a way, it will surpass the glorious Fioravanti.[10]
O Father Bacchus, O holy Bromius,
O Liber, O Dionysus, O great Lenaeus,
Pincerna and Canevar of the Aonian class,[11]
Give power to the great frenzy of my brain
With a glass well-filled with your Lyaeus
That would honor a new Orpheus.
You, Muses, who are wont to weave the acts of heroes
At the bobbin and spindle,
For now, go to the woods of Montello.[12]

---

[5] archlute.
[6] clapper: the giant Morgante's weapon in Pulci's romance.
[7] "Pedrala and Togna." In *Il Baldo*, Merlin Cocai (the pseudonym of Teofilo Folengo) rejects the traditional Muses and turns instead for his inspiration to his "macaronic muses," the countrywomen Berta, Gosaque, Togna, Simul, Mofelina, Pedrala, and Convina. They feed him on gnocchi. See *Partitiol: Le opere maccheroniche di Merlin Cocai* (Mantua: Mondovi, 1882).
[8] Merlin Cocai, popular writer of macaronic pieces. See above.
[9] Gradella: Commedia dell'Arte character. See p. 112, note 16.
[10] Fioravanti: See p. 52, note 49.
[11] "Bromius ... Canevar," all epithets for Bacchus, god of wine.
[12] Montello: woods about 10 miles north of Treviso.

To Angelucci: In Praise of Madness

In madness, I can sing—just as well without you—
Of the humors and frenzies
That reside in all our brains.
What singing is more pleasant than that on madness,
A topic so widespread in the world
That it deserves praise and honor in a thousand ways?
See how high the material rises
So that chaos—the first compound—
Took its name from matter.
Furthermore, that motion to which the world was exposed
Is here a clear and obvious dignity;
It was also presented as an Idea to the crazy brain.
The celestial worlds have expressly
Within them a variety of matter,
As they move towards their setting in the west.
All the spheres have such a pattern in them
That they spin in circles as if crazy.
In this they resemble a vacuous brain.
The stars are swept along by the firmament
Just as a foolish act is executed by
A racing brain faster than the swiftest barge.
The more I lift myself up with my thinking and advance
Myself inside, the more I see, and understand
The true and veritable core of the matter.
The Primum Mobile, being so fast,
Resembles a fantastic humor,
And a brain that is always racing.
The eighth sphere has this marvel:
That, trembling, it races like a madman
Who is constantly batting his eyelashes out of fear.
And the moon shows, in its behavior,
That it has great sympathy with lunatics,
Who always have their brains upside down.
Saturn fills them with melancholy,
And Mars does its job very well
With some influences full of oddity.
A madman holds the entire universe with its spheres
Inside his head, and he demonstrates
How it corresponds with his own brain.
Because it prepares him to be changeable
And almost continuously brings
The Tropic and Cancer constellation into his head.
The brawny humor leads him from one pole to the other;

In a moment, and with swift thinking,
He hops from pillar to post by the shortest route.
But the whole world will say with one voice
That a madman is like a wise man in every other way.
Nor can what I have said harm his reputation
Because it is well known that such a humor
Was not done properly,
Nor was a brain that has leap-year sculpted on its top.
I, without fail, will also try this trick,
Providing my brain will not go north
But will stay in its proper place, where it has now stopped.
Because, were it to get off its track,
It would be impossible to carry out such an enterprise
Without wrapping a foot of cable around its neck,
Though it would not be something new,
Because sometimes it sails so fast
That it reaches the antipodes in an instant.
Is there anyone who does not at times wear it
On his beret? And does it not fly with his thoughts
Faster even than a courier?
Now we can clearly see whether a fool steals
Virtue from wisdom.
He does not spend his sleeping hours under the bedsheets.
On the contrary, he cares so much about proving to be good
In the arts and sciences that he studies all day,
And allowing his brain to rest is a thing most loathsome to him.
He is so adorned with Mathematics
That he seems to steal his name from it
And carries it like an honor, not for scorn.
Arithmetic seems to produce worthy results
In him, since he can always count
How many phantasms a barn owl understands.
Geometry honors him and makes him illustrious, as well,
Because without using a compass or a sextant
He measures his follies hour by hour.
In music he appears a giant,
And while he hardly knows the gamut[13]
He is loud enough, if he wants, to be heard in the East.
But if he knew from A-la to C-ut,
He would make such a mess of Giachette

---

[13] gamut: the musical hexachord.

That he would reduce him to a *ceffaut*.[14]
If he sometimes dedicates himself to astrology
He can go on astrologizing for more than a month,
As if he was the king of owls.
Often he sets his eyes on philosophy,
And more than anything else, he understands the void,
And, even more, chaos, because that's what he has learned the best.
Sometimes he even ventures into logic,
And syllogizing, he often concludes
That his knowledge can rival that of donkeys.
In grammar he runs with naked legs
And with rhetoric like a cuckoo's
He shows Fidentio, whether he is erudite or rude.[15]
And, though his head is made of plaster
He knows the Code and the Digest,[16]
And in disputing he seems to be playing tricks.
But don't assume that, since he is expert in this,
He does not understand anything else either,
Since he is more skilled in the commentary than in the text.
Go ahead, turn him around from stem to stern, if you know how,
For he knows how to raise a mast properly,
And how to sail on constantly with that little brain of his.
This is what pertains to his glories,
But he has privileges in many other things,
More numerous than all the owls of Athens.
A madman certainly has a better time than kings
Or emperors ever had on earth,
And all of Madness is full of ornaments
As long as the breadbox is open.
He does not care for delicacies, or treats,
Nor for sugar-coated *zabaglione*.[17]
He does not seek cakes, or roasted livers.
He does not care for sausages from Modena,
Nor for all the broths of Milan, or for delicacies.

---

[14] "ceffaut," a contraction of "Ce-Sol-Fa-Ut," meaning a fractured or ruined scale or music. This madman would corrupt the wonderful music of Giaches de Wert (Jacquet of Mantua) and turn it into cacophony.

[15] Fidentio: the author of popular macaronic verse, *I cantici di Fidentio Glottogrysio Ludimagistro* (Florence, 1574).

[16] Roman law of Justinian.

[17] zabaglione: a dessert with heavy whipped cream flavored with marsala or other sweet wine.

If he spites the kitchen in his heart
He also does not care much for the cellar,
For a sip of water to him is a royal drink.
He cares as much for going to bed dressed
As for being naked among clothed people,
And as much for the evening as for daybreak.
It makes no difference to him whether his food is undigested or raw,
Or if he has good digestion;
For he is free and naked of all passions.
You never see him argue with others
Like some do, for the sake of money.
Nor will he ever sell his coat to go gambling.
He will not spend a cent on fights,
And in things pertaining to the palace of Mainardo
You will not be able to get even a morsel from him.
If you look at acts of justice,
In all his things he is so honest
He is like a kidney that never embraced lard.
On the contrary, he plays so clean
That he has no fear of policemen or torturers,
And he does not think much of their positions.
A madman does not look for, nor does he obtain, advice
When he has the law at his heels,
And everything he does he does at random.
He does not pay any attention to his savings,
Unlike some sugar-coated shits [18]
Who eat spiders instead of capons.
He has all his acts well regulated within himself.
He lives merrily and without worries,
Despite there being so many desperate people.
He does not need to think of what he will do this year,
Nor if there is going to be feast or famine,
Or if the harvests will be good or bad.
He does not have to worry, and is not inclined to accumulate
Money, the way greedy people—who
Deserve the evil they get from God—do.
Madmen are so simple and good
That they are outside the herd of hypocrites
And parasites.
Because their minds are not so wicked,

---

[18] "sugar-coated shits," *stronzi confettati*: said of those who are undeservedly praised.

The way others are, like those who have a wry-neck[19]
Or go to the tavern to have fun with the ribald crowd.
Regarding matters of the world, they are as if dead,
And so dull, that the poor souls
Are easily identified both in their goodness and their evil.
But if they are inept in these dealings
Their simplicity ought to be praised
For it gives birth to most useful effects.
You will never find a madman selling you
Bread made with dust, the way a baker would,
Or one who spends other people's money and steals it.
He will not wage war against you with violence and hatred,
Nor will he get the Lord's mule pregnant,
The way that clever one from Volterra did.
He may not sing the Miserere like others;
He will not tell stories or lies,
Nor will he relate fables as if they were true;
He will not reveal other people's sins
The way some wily, clever people do,
Always seeking discord and trouble.
But even with such beautiful attributes,
Madness is criticized by many people
Whom the populace considers to have decent brains.
As for myself, I have praised it as it deserves,
And I criticize completely that unjust school
That has tormented it through unworthy writings.
Now may they be hanged by their necks!

---

[19] "wry-neck," from excessive bowing, either in church or at court.

Bibliography

Primary Sources

Aelianus, Claudius. *Historia varia*. Trans. Diane Ostrom Johnson. Lewiston: Mellen Press, 1997.

———. *Historical Miscellany*. Trans. Nigel Wilson. Loeb Classical Library. Cambridge, MA: Harvard University Press, 1997.

———. *On the Characteristics of Animals*. Trans. A.F. Scholfield. 3 vols. Loeb Classical Library. Cambridge, MA: Harvard University Press, 1958.

Aegineta, Paulus. *The Seven Books on Medicine*. Trans. Francis Adams. 3 vols. London: Sydenham Society, 1844–1847.

Aëtius of Amida. *Tetrabiblion*. Lyons: Beringorum, 1549.

Agrippa, Henricius Cornelius. *De incertitudine & vanitate omnium scientiarum*. Lyons: Matthaei, 1643.

Albergati, Vianesio. *La pazzia*. Venice: Giovanni Andrea Valvassori, 1541.

Alberti, Leon Battista. *Momus*. Ed. and trans. Sarah Knight. Cambridge, MA: Harvard University Press, 2004.

Alciato, Andrea. *Emblematum libellus nuper in lucem editus*. Venice: Sons of Aldo Manuzio, 1546.

Altomare, Donato. *De medendis humani corporis malis ars medica*. Naples: Cancer Mattia, 1553.

Ambianus, John Fernelius (Jean Fernel of Amiens). *Medicina*. Paris: André Wechel, 1554.

———. *The practice of physik in seventeen books…* . London: Streator, 1668.

Ambrose. *De Elia et ieiuno*. PL 14.697–728.

Angelucci, Teodoro. *Ars Medica ex Hippocratis Galenique thesauris potissimum deprompta*. Venice: Paolo Meietto, 1588.

Apollodorus. *The Library of Greek Mythology*. Trans. Robin Hard. New York: Oxford University Press, 1997.

Ariosto, Ludovico. *Orlando furioso*. Ferrara: Francesco Rosso of Valenza, 1532.

———. Trans. W.S. Rose, ed. Stuart A. Baker and A. Bartlett Giamatti. New York: Bobbs–Merrill, 1968.

———. *The Satires of Ludovico Ariosto: A Renaissance Biography*. Trans. P.D. Wiggins. Athens, OH: Ohio University Press, 1976.

Aristophanes. *The Frogs*. Trans. Richmond Lattimore. Ann Arbor: University of Michigan Press, 1962.

Aristotle. "Eudemian Ethics." In *The Athenian Constitution, The Eudemian Ethics on Virtues and Vices.* Trans. H. Rackham. Loeb Classical Library. Cambridge, MA: Harvard University Press, 1952.

Arlotto, Mainardi. *Facezie, fabule e motti del Piovano Arlotto.* Florence: Zucchetta, 1515.

———. *Motti e facezie del Piovano Arlotto.* Ed. Gianfranco Folena. Milan: Ricciardi, 1995.

Athenaeus. *Dipnosophistarum sive Coenae sapientium Libri XV.* Trans. Natale Conti. Venice: Andrea Arrivabene, 1556.

———. *The Deipnosophists.* Ed. and trans. Charles Breton Gulick. Loeb Classical Library. London: Putnam's, 1927.

Atti dei notai del comune di Bagnacavallo and *Governatori di Bagnacavallo.* State Archives of Ravenna.

Aulus Gellius. *The Attic Nights.* Trans. John C. Rolfe. Loeb Classical Library. Cambridge, MA: Harvard University Press, 1984.

Ausonius. *Ausonius.* Trans. H.G. Evelyn White. 2 vols. Loeb Classical Library. New York: Putnam's, 1919–1921.

Badius Ascensius, Jodocus. *Nauis stultifere collectanea.* Paris: J. Badius Ascensius and the de Marnef brothers, 1513. Grenoble: Université, 1979.

Bargagli, Scipione. *La prima parte dell'imprese.* Siena: Bonetti, 1578.

———. *Dell'imprese.* Venice: Francesco de'Franceschi, 1594.

Bembo, Pietro. *Gli Asolani.* Trans. Rudolf B. Gottfried. Bloomington: Indiana University Press, 1954.

Benivieni, Antonio. *De abditis nonnullis ac mirandis morborum et sanationum causis.* Florence: Filippo Giunta, 1507.

———. Ed. G. Weber. Florence: Olschki, 1994.

Brant, Sebastian. *The Ship of Fools.* Trans., intro. and comm. Edwin H. Zeydel. New York: Columbia University Press, 1944.

Brasavola, Antonio Musa. *Aphorismorum Hippocratis et Galeni commentaria et annotationes.* Basel: Officina Frobeniana, 1541.

Bugati, Gasparo. *Historia universale.* Venice: Giolito, 1571.

Burton, Robert. *The Anatomy of Melancholy.* Ed. and intro. Holbrook Jackson, intro. William H. Gass. New York: New York Review of Books, 2001.

———. Ed. T. C. Faulkner et al. Oxford: Clarendon Press, 1989.

[Celio] Ricchieri, Ludovico. *Lectionum antiquarum libri XXX.* Lyons: Sebastian Honorat, 1560.

Caburacci, Francesco. *Trattato di M. Francesco Caburacci da Imola. Dove si dimostra il vero, et il novo modo di fare le Imprese, con un breve discorso in difesa dell'Orlando Furioso di M. Ludovico Ariosto.* Bologna: Giovanni Rossi, 1580.

Capaccio, Giulio Cesare. *Delle imprese.* Naples: Gio. Giacomo Carlino and Antonio Pace, 1592.

Cato. *Disticha de moribus.* Paris: S. Stephanus, 1557.

Cicero. *On Oratory*. Trans. and ed. I.S. Watson, intro. Ralph A. Micken, David Potter, and Richard Leo Enos. Carbondale: Southern Illinois University Press, 1970.

———. *Letters to Friends*. Ed. and trans. D.R. Shackleton Bailey. Loeb Classical Library. Cambridge, MA: Harvard University Press, 2001.

———. *Verrines*. Trans. and comm. T.N. Mitchell. Atlantic Highlands, NJ: Aris & Phillips, 1986.

Claudian. *Claudian*. Trans. Maurice Platnauer. Loeb Classical Library. New York: Putnam's, 1922.

Conti, Natale, ed. and trans. *Athenaei Dipnosophistarum* . . . . Lyons: Faure, Jacques Honorat, Barthelemy, 1556.

Crinito, Pietro. *De honesta disciplina*. Ed. Carlo Angeleri. Rome: Bocca, 1955.

Dante. *Inferno*. Trans. and ed. Mark Musa. Bloomington: Indiana University Press, 1995.

———. *Purgatory*. Trans, notes and comm. Mark Musa. Bloomington: Indiana University Press, 1981.

Diodorus Siculus. *Diodorus of Sicily*. Trans. C.H. Oldfather. Loeb Classical Library. Cambridge, MA: Harvard University Press, 1935.

Diogenes Laertius. *Lives of Eminent Philosophers*. Trans. R.D. Hicks. Loeb Classical Library. Cambridge, MA: Harvard University Press, 1931–1938.

Dionysius the Carthusian. *Colloquio, overo dialogo del giudicio particolare dell'animo dopo la morte*. Trans. Tomaso Garzoni. Venice: Francesco Ziletti, 1583.

Doni, Anton Francesco. *I marmi del Doni, academico peregrino*. Venice: Francesco Marcolini, 1552.

Erasmus. *Moriae Encomium*. Basle: Frobenius, 1519.

———. *Adages*. Trans. Margaret Mann Phillips, annot. R.A.B. Mynors. 6 vols. Collected Works of Erasmus 31–36. Toronto and Buffalo: University of Toronto Press, 1982–2006.

Eusebius Pamphili. *Ecclesiastical History*. Trans. Roy J. Deferrari. New York: Fathers of the Church, 1953–1955.

———. *Chronici Canones*. Ed. John Knight Fotheringham. London: Humphrey Milford, 1818.

Eustathius. *Commentarii ad Homeri Odysseam*. Leipzig: Weigel, 1885; repr. Hildesheim: Olms, 1970.

Eutropius. *Abridgment of Roman History*. Trans. John Selby Watson. London: Henry G. Bohn, 1853.

Farra, Alessandro. *Settenario dell'humana riduttione*. Venice: Christoforo Zanetti, 1571.

Fernel. See Ambianus.

Fioravanti, Leonardo. *An exact collection of the choicest and more rare experiments and secrets in physick and chyrurgery (both chymick and Galenick) viz. of Leonard Phioravant* . . . London: William Shears, 1659.

Folegno, Teofilo (ps. Merlin Cocai). *Il Baldus*. In *Le opere maccheroniche di Merlin Cocai*. Mantua: Mondovi, 1882–1889.

Galluccio, Luigi (called Elisio Calenzio). *Epigrammata*. In *Opuscula Elisii Calentii poetae clarissimi . . . Epigrammaton libellus*. Rome: Ioannes de Besicken, 1503.

Garzoni, Bartolomeo. "Laconismo vitale circa l'autore." In Tomaso Garzoni, *Il serraglio de gli stupori del mondo* . . . . Venice: Bartolomeo Dei, 1613.

———, and Tomaso Garzoni. *Gli due Garzoni, cioè l'huomo astratto del molto rever. P. D. Tomaso Garzoni da Bagnacavallo; & la stella de' magi del molto rever. P. D. Bartolomeo Garzoni da Bagnacavallo, amendue fratelli per natura, per studio, per religione, per titolo di predicatore o teologo, et per nominatione d'academici, in varie città d'Italia*. Venice: G.B. Ciotti Senese, 1604.

Garzoni, Tomaso. *Il theatro de' vari e diversi cervelli mondani*. Venice: Paulo Zanfretti, 1583.

———. *L'hospidale de' pazzi incurabili . . . nuovamente formato, & posto in luce da Tomaso Garzoni da Bagnacauallo Con tre capitoli in fine sopra la pazzia*. Ferrara: Giulio Cesare Cagnacini & Brothers, 1586; Venice: G.B. Somasco, 1586.

———. *L'hospidale de pazzi incurabili . . . Aggiontoui di nouo due copiosissime tauole . . .* Piacenza: Giovanni Bazachi, 1586.

———. *La piazza universale di tutte le professioni del mondo, e nobili et ignobili*. Venice: G.B.Somasco, 1586.

———. Ed. Paolo Cherchi and Beatrice Collina. Turin: Einaudi, 1996.

———. *Le vite delle donne illustri, e laide delle Sacre Scritture*. Venice: Domenico Imberti, 1586.

———. *La sinagoga de gl'ignoranti*. Venice: G.B Somasco, 1589.

———. *Il mirabile cornucopia consolatorio*. Bologna: Heirs of Giovanni Rossi, 1601.

———. *Il serraglio de gli stupori del mondo…arricchita di varie annotazioni dal M.R. P. D. Bartolomeo Garzoni suo fratello …* Venice: Bartolomeo Dei, 1613.

Giovio, Paolo. *Historiarum sui temporis libri II*. Florence: Torrentini, 1550–1552.

Giraldi, Lilio Gregorio. *Historia de deis gentium*. Basel: Joannes Oporinus, 1548; facs. repr. New York: Garland, 1976.

———. *De deis gentium libri sive syntagmata XVII [. . .]*. Lyons: Haeredes Iacobi Iunctae, 1565.

———. *Opera omnia*. Leiden: Hackius, 1696.

Gratian. *The Treatise on Laws : Decretum*. Trans. Augustine Thompson. Washington, DC: Catholic University of America Press, 1993.

Herodotus. *Histories*. Trans. A.D. Godley. Loeb Classical Library. Cambridge, MA: Harvard University Press, 1957.

Hesiod. *Theogony*. Trans. with intro. and notes M.L. West. New York: Oxford University Press, 1988.

Hippocrates. *The Aphorisms of Hippocrates and the Sentences of Celsus* .... London: Bonwick, 1708.
Homer. *The Iliad*. Trans. with intro. Richmond Lattimore. Chicago: University of Chicago Press, 1961.
Horace. *Odes and Epodes*. Trans. with intro. and comm. David Mulroy. Ann Arbor: University of Michigan Press, 1994.
———. *Satires, Epistles and Ars poetica*. Trans. H. Rushton Fairclough. Loeb Classical Library. New York: Putnam's, 1929.
Horapollo. *Ori Apollinis Niliaci, de sacris Aegyptiorum notis, Aegyptiace expressis libri duo, iconibus illustratis et auctis. Nunc primum in Latinum ac Gallicum sermonem conversi*. Paris: Galliot du Pré, 1574.
Hugh of Saint Victor. *Hugonis de Sancto Victore, Canonici Regularis Lateranensis, tum pietate, tum doctrina insignis, Opera tribus tomis digesta. Nunc a donno Thoma Garzonio de Bagnacaballo postillis, annotatiunculis, scholijs, ac vita auctoris expolita*. Venice: G.B. Somasco, 1588.
Jacobus de Voragine. *The Golden Legend: Readings on the Saints*. Trans. William Granger Ryan. 2 vols. Princeton: Princeton University Press, 1993.
Juvenal. *Satires*. In *Juvenal and Persius*. Trans. S.M. Braund. Loeb Classical Library. Cambridge, MA: Harvard University Press, 2004.
Kühn, C.G., ed. *Medicorum graecorum opera quae exstant*. Leipzig: Knobloch, 1821–1833.
Lando, Ortensio. *Sette libri di cathaloghi a varie cose appartenenti, non solo antiche, ma anche moderne*. Ferrara: Gabriel Giolito de Ferrari, 1552.
Leoni, Domenico. *Ars medendi humanos*. Bologna: Giovanni Rossi, 1583.
Lucan. *The Civil War: Pharsalia*. Trans. J.D. Duff. Loeb Classical Library. Cambridge, MA: Harvard University Press, 1977.
Lucian. *Lucian*. Trans. A.M. Harmon. Loeb Classical Library. Cambridge, MA: Harvard University Press, 1960.
———. "Timon the Misanthrope." In *The Works of Lucian of Samosata*, trans. H.W. Fowler and L.G. Fowler. Oxford: Clarendon Press, 1905.
[Lucilius.] In *Incerti auctoris Aetna*. Ed. with intro and comm. F.R.D. Goodyear. Cambridge: Cambridge University Press, 1965.
Lull, Raymond. *Obras*. Ed. with notes Jerónimo Rosselló. Palma de Mallorca: Hijas de Colomar, 1901–1903.
Manuzio, Paolo. *Adagia*. Florence: Apud Iuntas, 1575.
Orologi, Giuseppe. *L'inganno*. Venice: Gabriele Giolito de' Ferrari, 1562.
Ovid. *The Art of Love*. Trans. James Michie, intro. David Malouf. New York: Modern Library, 2002.
———. *The Fasti, Tristia, Pontic Epistles, Ibis, and Halieuticon*. Trans. H.T. Riley. London: George Bell, 1879.
———. *Metamorphoses*. Trans. Frank Justus Miller. 2 vols. Loeb Classical Library. Cambridge, MA: Harvard University Press, 1984.

———. *Opere di Publio Ovidio Nasone*. Ed. Francesco Della Corte and Silvana Fasce. Turin: Unione Tipografico, 1986.
Pausanias. *Description of Greece*. Trans. W.H. Jones and H.A. Ormerod. Loeb Classical Library. Cambridge, MA: Harvard University Press, 1918.
———. *Guide to Greece*. Trans. Peter Levi. Harmondsworth: Penguin, 1979.
Petrarca, Francesco. *Le cose volgari de Messer Francesco Petrarcha*. Venice: Aldo Manuzio, 1501.
———. *Canzoniere*. Trans. Mark Musa, intro. idem and Barbara Manfredi. Bloomington: Indiana University Press, 1996.
———. "The Triumph of Time." In *Triumphs*, trans. E.H. Wilkins. Chicago: University of Chicago Press, 1962.
Petrus Hispanus. *Language in Dispute: An English Translation of Peter of Spain's Tractatus, called afterwards Summulae Logicales*. Trans. Francis P. Dinneed. Philadelphia: Benjamins, 1990.
Philostratus. In *Philostratus and Eunapius, The Lives of the Sophists*. Trans. W.C.F. Wright. Loeb Classical Library. New York: Putnam's, 1922.
Plato. *Theaetetus*. Trans. R.A.H. Waterfield. New York: Viking Penguin, 1987.
Pliny the Elder. *Natural History*. Trans. H. Rackham. Loeb Classical Library. Cambridge, MA: Harvard University Press, 1949.
Pliny the Younger. *Letters*. Trans. William Melmoth, rev. W.M.L. Hutchinson. New York: Macmillan, 1915.
Plutarch. *Lives*. Trans. B. Perrin. New York: Macmillan, 1914–1926.
———. *Moralia*. Trans. Frank Cole Bobbitt. 15 vols. Loeb Classical Library. Cambridge, MA: Harvard University Press, 1962.
Poliziano, Angelo. *Angeli Politiani Silva cui titulus Nutricia*. Florence: Antonius Misconminos, 1485.
———. Trans. and ed. C. Fantazzi. Cambridge, MA: Harvard University Press, 2004.
———. *Poesie italiane*. Ed. Salverio Orlando, intro. Mario Luzi. Milan: Rizzoli, 1998.
Possevino, Antonio. *Bibliotheca selecta qua agitur de ratione studiorum in historia, in disciplinis, in salute omnium procuranda*. 2 vols. Rome: Dominicus Basa, 1593.
———. *Apparatus sacer ad scriptores veteris, & novi Testamenti*. 3 vols. Venice: Società Veneta, 1603.
Priscianus, Theodorus. *Rerum medicarum libri quatuor*. Strasbourg: Joannes Schottus, 1532.
Propertius. *Elegies*. Ed. and trans. G.P. Goold. Loeb Classical Library. Cambridge, MA: Harvard University Press, 1990.
Pseudo–Aristotle. *Secretum secretorum*. Lyons: Antoine Blanchard, 1528.
———. *Mirabilia*. Ed. and trans. Hellmut Flashar and Ulrich Klein. Berlin: Akademie–Verlag, 1990.

Pulci, Luigi. *Morgante: The Epic Adventures of Orlando and his Giant Friend Morgante*. Trans. Joseph Tusiani, intro. and notes Edoardo A. Lèbano. Bloomington: Indiana University Press, 1998.
Ruscelli, Girolamo. *Le imprese illustri*. Venice: Francesco Rampazetto, 1566.
———. *Sopplimento di Girolamo Ruscelli nell'Historie di Monsignor Paolo Giovio*. Venetia: Silicato, 1572.
Sallust. *The Jugurthine War and The Conspiracy of Catiline*. Trans. S.A. Handford. Baltimore: Penguin, 1963.
Scriptores Historiae Augustae. Trans. David Magie. Loeb Classical Library. Cambridge, MA: Harvard University Press, 1967.
Seneca. *Epistles*. Trans. R.M. Gummere. Loeb Classical Library. New York: Putnam's, 1925.
———. *Phaedra*. Ed. Michael Coffey and Roland Mayer. New York: Cambridge University Press, 1990.
Seneca the Elder. *Controversiae*. Trans. M. Winterbottom. Loeb Classical Library. Cambridge, MA: Harvard University Press, 1974.
Silius Italicus. *Punica*. Trans. J.D. Duff. Loeb Classical Library. Cambridge, MA: Harvard University Press, 1934.
Strabo. *The Geography of Strabo*. Trans. H.L. Jones. Loeb Classical Library. Cambridge, MA: Harvard University Press, 1960.
Strozzi, Tito Vespasiano. *Eroticon*. In *Strozzi poetae pater et filivs*. Basle: Westhemer, 1545.
Suetonius. *Suetonius*. Trans. J.C. Rolfe. Loeb Classical Library. Cambridge, MA: Harvard University Press, 1997.
Tacitus. *The Histories*. Trans. Clifford H. Morre. Loeb Classical Library. New York: Putnam's, 1925–1937.
Tasso, Torquato. *Aminta, fauola boscareccia*. Venice: Aldo Manuzio the Younger, 1580.
Terence. *The Eunuch*. Ed. with trans. and comm. A.J. Brothers. Warminster: Aris & Phillips, 2000.
Tesauro, Emanuele. *Idea delle perfette imprese*. Ed. M.L. Doglio. Florence: Olschki, 1975.
Theobald. *Physiologus*. Trans. Alan Wood Rendell. London: Bumpus, 1928.
Tixier de Ravisy, Jean. *Officina*. Basel: Nikolaus Brylinger, 1552.
Valeriano, Pierio Bolzano. *Hieroglyphica sive de sacris Aegyptiorum literis commentarii*. Basle: Michael Isengrin, 1556.
Valerius Maximus. *Memorable Doings and Sayings*. Trans. D.R. Shackleton Bailey. Loeb Classical Library. Cambridge, MA: Harvard University Press, 2000.
Virgil. *The Aeneid*. Trans. David West. New York: Penguin, 1990.
———. *Bucolics*. In *The Eclogues, Bucolics, or Pastorals of Virgil*. Trans. T.F. Royds. Oxford: Blackwell, 1922.

Bibliography: Secondary Works

Anonymous, ed. *Tomaso Garzoni: Un zingaro in convento. Celebrazioni garzoniane, IV centenario 1589–1989, Ravenna–Bagnacavallo 1989–1990.* Ravenna: Longo, 1990.
Avesani, Remo. "La professione dell' 'umanista' nel Cinquecento." *Italia medievale e umanistica* 13 (1970): 205–32.
Baruchello, François. "Tomaso Garzoni, precursore della psichiatria moderna." In *Tomaso Garzoni: Un zingaro in convento*, 179–204.
Bernardini, Franca Fedeli, ed. *L'ospedale dei pazzi di Roma dai papi al '900: Lineamenti di assistenza e cura a poveri e dementi.* Vol. 2. Rome: Dedalo, 1994.
———. " 'Il vasto casamento della romana misericordia': Note per una storia delle istituzioni assistenziali nella Roma post–tridentina." In *L'ospedale dei pazzi di Roma*, ed. eadem, 2:273–78.
Bernardis, Alberto de, ed. *Follia, psichiatria e società: Istituzioni manicomiali, scienza psichiatrica e classi sociali nell' Italia moderna e contemporanea.* Milan: Angeli, 1982.
Biondi, Albano. "Aspetti della cultura cattolica post–tridentina: Religione e controllo sociale." In *Storia d'Italia, Annali* 4: *Intellettuali e potere*, ed. C. Vivanti, 253–302. Turin: Einaudi, 1981.
Biotti, Vittorio. "Il folle nella società fiorentina e toscana del XVI e XVII sec. e la nascita di 'S. Dorotea de' Pazzarelli'." In *Follia, psichiatria e società*, ed. de Bernardis, 170–210.
Blair, Ann. *The Theater of Nature: Jean Bodin and Renaissance Science.* Princeton: Princeton University Press, 1997.
Bolzoni, Lina. *Il teatro della memoria: Studi su G. Camillo.* Padua: Liviana, 1984.
———. *La stanza della memoria.* Turin: Einaudi, 1995.
———. "Come costruire il tesoro della memoria: La tradizione mnemotecnica." In *Ricerche sulle selve rinascimentali*, ed. P. Cherchi, 157–73. Ravenna: Longo, 1999.
Bonella, Anna Lia, ed. *L'ospedale dei pazzi di Roma dai papi al '900: Fonti per la storia della follia. Santa Maria della Pietà e il suo archivio storico sec. XVI–XX.* Vol. 1. Rome: Dedalo, 1994.
Bonfigli, Alessandra, and Franca Fedeli Bernardini. " 'Quella carità che si sol fare alli pazzi acciò venghi a recuperare la sanità': Gli esordi dell' ospedale di S. Maria della Pietà e la cura dei dementi." In *L'ospedale dei pazzi di Roma*, ed. Bernardini, 2:41–56.
Bonfil, Robert. *English Jewish Life in Renaissance Italy.* Trans. Anthony Oldcorn. Berkeley: University of California Press, 1994.
Borsetto, Luciana. *Il furto di Prometeo: Imitazione, scrittura, riscrittura nel Rinascimento.* Alessandria: Edizioni dell' Orso, 1990.
Brumble, H. David. *Classical Myths and Legends in the Middle Ages and Renaissance.* Westport, CT: Greenwood Press, 1998.

Bylebyl, Jerome. "Medicine, Philosophy, Humanism in Renaissance Italy." In *Science and the Arts in the Renaissance*, ed. John W. Shirley and David Hoeniger, 27–49. London and Toronto: Associated University Presses, 1985.

Calabritto, Monica. "The Subject of Madness: An Analysis of Ariosto's *Orlando Furioso* and Garzoni's *L'hospedale de' pazzi incurabili*." Ph.D diss., City University of New York, 2001.

———. "Garzoni's *L' hospedale de' pazzi incurabili* and the Ambiguous Relation between Word and Image in Sixteenth–century *impresa*." *Emblematica* 13 (2003): 97–130.

Caldwell, Dorigen. "The *paragone* between Word and Image in *imprese* Literature." *Journal of the Warburg and Courtauld Institutes* 63 (2000): 277–86.

———. "Studies in the Sixteenth–century Italian *impresa*." *Emblematica* 11 (2001): 1–257.

———. *The Sixteenth–Century Impresa in Theory and Practice*. New York: AMS Press, 2004.

Cherchi, Paolo. "'In bus e in bas'." *Lingua Nostra* 29 (1968): 108.

———. "La grazia di S. Paolo." *Lingua Nostra* 30 (1969): 120.

———. "L'encomio paradossale nel manierismo." *Forum Italicum* 9 (1975): 368–84.

———. *Enciclopedismo e politica della riscrittura: Tomaso Garzoni*. Pisa: Pacini, 1980.

———. "L' *Officina* del Testore e alcune opere di Ortensio Lando." *Modern Language Notes* 95 (1980): 210–19.

———. "Introduzione." In Tomaso Garzoni, *Opere*, ed. idem, 7–22. Ravenna: Longo, 1993.

———. "Invito alla lettura della Piazza." In Tomaso Garzoni, *La piazza universale di tutte le professioni del mondo*, ed. idem and B. Collina, XXI–LXVI. Turin: Einaudi, 1996.

———. ed. *Sondaggi sulla riscrittura del Cinquecento*. Ravenna: Longo, 1998.

———. "La selva rinascimentale: profilo di un genere." In *Ricerche sulle selve rinascimentali*, ed. idem, 9–41. Ravenna: Longo, 1999.

———. "T. Garzoni, bestseller europeo: perché?" In *Tomaso Garzoni: Uno zingaro in convento*, 109–123.

Clark, Stuart. *Thinking with Demons: The Idea of Witchcraft in Early Modern Europe*. New York: Oxford University Press, 1997.

Collina, Beatrice. "Un 'cervello universale'." In Garzoni, *La piazza universale di tutte le professioni del mondo*, ed. P. Cherchi and eadem, LXVII–CVII.

———. "Introduction." In Tomaso Garzoni, *Le vite delle donne illustri, e laide delle Sacre Scritture*, ed. eadem, 7–71. Ravenna: Longo, 1994.

Cracco, Giorgio, ed. *Nuovi Studi Ezzeliniani*. 2 vols. Rome: Istituto Palazzo Borromini, 1992.

Dictionnaire des Sciences Médicales: Biographie Médicale. 7 vols. Paris: Panckoucke, 1820–1825.

Di Francia, Letterio. *Novellistica*. Milan: Vallardi, 1925.
Dizionario biografico degli italiani. Rome: Istituto della Enciclopedia Italiana. 1960–.
Dizionario degli Istituti di perfezione. Rome: Edizioni Paoline, 1974–2003.
Ferretti, Giuseppe. "L'umanista Tomaso Garzoni, religioso e scrittore Bagnacavallese nel quarto centenario della morte." *Torricelliana: Bollettino della società torricelliana di scienze e lettere* 41 (1990): 191–200.
Ferri, Luigi. *Vocabulario ferrarese–italiano*. Bologna: Forni, 1967.
Ferro, Filippo Maria. "Il gran teatro della Romana pietà." In *L'ospedale dei pazzi di Roma*, ed. Bernardini, 2:27–39.
Fiorato, Adelin Charles. "La folie universelle, spectacle burlesque et instrument idéologique dans *L'hospedale* de Tomaso Garzoni (1586)." In *Visages de la folie (1500–1600): Colloque tenu à la Sorbonne le 8 et le 9 mai*, ed. A. Redondo and A. Rochon, 131–45. Paris: Publications de la Sorbonne, 1981.
Foa, Anna. *Ebrei in Europa: Dalla peste all'emancipazione*. Bari: Laterza, 1997.
Gager, John G. *The Origins of Anti-Semitism: Attitudes toward Judaism in Pagan and Christian Antiquity*. New York: Oxford University Press, 1983.
Garzoni, Tomaso. *L'hospidale del pazzi incurabili*. Ed. Stefano Barelli. Rome: Antenore, 2004.
——. *L'hospital des fols incurables*. Trans. François de Clarier, ed. and intro. A.C. Fiorato. Paris: Champion; Geneva: Slatkine, 2001.
——. *Le vite delle donne illustri, e laide delle Sacre Scritture*. Ed. Beatrice Collina. Ravenna: Longo, 1994.
——. *Il serraglio de gli stupori del mondo…arricchita di varie annotazioni dal M.R. P. D. Bartolomeo Garzoni suo fratello*. Intro. Paolo Cerchi. Ravenna: Russi, 2004.
——. *Opere*. Ed. Paolo Cherchi. Ravenna: Longo, 1993.
Gerbino, Giuseppe. "The Madrigal and its Outcasts: Marenzio, Giovannelli, and the Revival of Sannazaro's *Arcadia*." *Journal of Musicology* 21 (2004): 29–31.
Giorio, Elvinia Vidali. "Una fonte del Garzoni: Dello specchio di scientia universale di Leonardo Fioravanti." *Lingua Nostra* 30 (1969): 39–43.
Gregory, Timothy. *Vox Populi: Popular Opinion and Violence in the Religious Controversies of the Fifth Century A.D.* Columbus, OH: Ohio State University Press, 1986.
Henderson, John. *The Renaissance Hospital: Healing the Body and Healing the Soul*. New Haven: Yale University Press, 2006.
Jourdan, A.L.J. *Biographie médicale*, suppl. to *Dictionaire des sciences médicales*. Paris: Panckoucke, 1820–1825.
Klein, Robert. "La théorie de l'expression figurée dans les traités italiens sur les *imprese*, 1555–1621." *Bibliothèque d'Humanisme et Renaissance* 19 (1957): 320–41.

Lea, K.M. *Italian Popular Comedy: A Study in the Commedia dell'arte, 1560–1620, with Special Reference to the English Stage.* Oxford: Clarendon Press, 1934.

Liruti, Gian Giuseppe. *Notizie delle vite ed opere scritte da letterati del Friuli.* Bologna: Forni, 1971.

Lo Schiavo, D. Luigi. "Tomaso Garzoni C.R.L. e la sua congregazione (1549–1589)." In *Tomaso Garzoni: Uno zingaro in convento*, 27–34.

Luzzati, Michele, Michele Olivari, and Alessandra Veronese, eds. *Ebrei e cristiani nell'Italia medievale e moderna: conversioni, scambi, contrasti: atti del VI congresso internazionale dell'AISG, S. Miniato, 4–6 novembre 1986.* Rome: Carucci, 1988.

Maggi, Armando. *Identità e impresa rinascimentale.* Ravenna: Longo, 1998.

———. *Satan's Rhetoric: A Study of Renaissance Demonology.* Chicago: University of Chicago Press, 2001.

———. "The Concept of 'natural ecstasy' in Tomaso Garzoni's *L'huomo astratto*." *Modern Philology* 101 (2003): 259–77.

Marchetti, Valerio. "La rappresentazione della follia: una biblioteca senza archivio." In *La follia, la norma, l'archivio: Prospettive storiografiche e orientamenti archivistici*, ed. M. Galzigna, 135–69. Venice: Marsilio, 1984.

———. "Tassonomie, citazioni, esempi e luoghi comuni." In *Tomaso Garzoni: Polyhistorismus und Interkulturalität in der frühen Neuzeit*, ed. Italo Michele Battafarano, 9–25. Bern: Peter Lang, 1991.

Mazzacurati, Giancarlo, and Michel Plaisance, eds. *Scritture di riscritture: Testi, generi, modelli nel Rinascimento.* Rome: Bulzoni, 1987.

Midelfort, Erik H.C. *A History of Madness in Sixteenth–Century Germany.* Stanford: Stanford University Press, 1999.

Mignon, Maurice. *Études sur le théatre français et italien de la Renaissance.* Paris: Champion, 1923.

Mulsow, Martin. "Ambiguities of the *Prisca Sapientia* in Late Renaissance Humanism." *Journal of the History of Ideas* 65 (2004): 1–13.

Ong, Walter. "Commonplace Rhapsody: Ravisius Textor, Zwinger and Shakespeare." In *Classical Influences on European Culture 1500–1700: Proceedings of an International Conference held at King's College, Cambridge, April 1974*, 91–126. Cambridge: Cambridge University Press, 1976.

Ossola, Carlo. "Métaphore et inventaire de la folie dans la littérature italienne du XVIe siècle." In *Folie et déraison à la Renaissance: Colloque international tenu en novembre 1973 sous les auspices de la Fédération Internationale des Instituts et Sociétés pour l'étude de la Renaissance*, 171–96. Brussels: Editions de l'Université de Bruxelles, 1976.

Oxford Dictionary of the Christian Church. 3rd ed. rev. Oxford: Oxford University Press, 1997.

Padovani, Giorgio. " 'L'hospidale de' pazzi incurabili' di Tomaso Garzoni: Una descrizione cinquecentesca delle principali forme di alienazione mentale." *Rassegna di Studi Psichiatrici* 38 (1943): 217–29.

Praz, Mario. *Studies in Seventeenth–Century Imagery*. 2 vols. London: The Warburg Institute, 1939–1947.

Prosperi, Adriano. "La Chiesa e gli ebrei nell'Italia del '500." In *Ebraismo e antiebraismo: immagine e pregiudizio*, 171–83. Florence: Giuntina, 1989.

Roger, Jacques. *Jean Fernel et les problèmes de la médicine de la Renaissance*. Paris: Palais de la Découverte, 1960.

Sangiorgi, Ada. Copies of manuscript document in possession of Monica Calabritto.

Savarese, Gennaro, and Andrea Gareffi, eds. *La letteratura delle immagini nel Cinquecento*. Rome: Bulzoni, 1980.

Scarpellini, Angelo. "Erasmo e i letterati Romagnoli del Cinquecento." *Studi Romagnoli* 18 (1967): 369–90.

Screech, M. A. "Good Madness in Christendom." In *The Anatomy of Madness: Essays in the History of Psychiatry*, vol. 1: *People and Ideas*, ed. W. F. Bynum, Roy Porter, and M. Shepherd, 25–39. London and New York: Tavistock Publications, 1985.

Seznec, Jean. *The Survival of the Pagan Gods*. Trans. Barbara F. Sessions. Princeton: Princeton University Press, 1972.

Simonini, Ivan. "Tomaso Garzoni, uno zingaro in convento." In *Tomaso Garzoni: uno zingaro in convento*, 9–25.

Siraisi, Nancy. *Avicenna in Renaissance Italy: The Canon and Medical Teaching in Italian Universities after 1500*. Princeton: Princeton University Press, 1987.

———. *The Clock and the Mirror: Girolamo Cardano and Renaissance Medicine*. Princeton: Princeton University Press, 1997.

Smith, William, ed. *Dictionary of Greek and Roman Biography and Mythology*. Boston: Little Brown, 1867.

Vodoz, Jules. *Le théatre latin de Ravisius Textor (1470–1524)*. Wintherthur: Imprimerie G. Ziegler, 1898.

Watson, Donald Gwynn. "Erasmus' *Praise of Folly* and the Spirit of Carnival." *Renaissance Quarterly* 32 (1979): 333–53.

Yates, Frances. *The Art of Memory*. Chicago: University of Chicago Press, 1984.

Index of Names

A

Abano, Pietro d', 130
Abila, 180
Abstemius, 42, 74
Abydos, 177
Acesias, 93–94
Achelous, 180
Acheron, 156
Achilles, 37, 78, 144, 157, 203
Adige, 58, 87
Admetus, King, 69, 180
Adrastia, 107
Adrastus, 107
Adriatic Sea, 85
Aeacus, 171
Aegean Sea, 90
Aegina, 56, 171
Aegineta, 17, 225
Aegiuchus, 65
Aelian, 87, 117–18, 121, 145, 177, 194, 196
Aelianus, 48, 225
Aeneas, 45, 64, 115, 133, 144, 184, 196
Aeolus, 158
Aeria, 119
Aeschylus, 113
Aesclepius, 37
Aesop, 124, 139, 191, 194
Aëtius, 55, 61, 63
Aetna, 144, 183, 186
Aetolia, King of, 180
Africa, 158
Agamemnon, 159
Agathyrses, 47
Agave, 159
Agesilaus, 72
Agoracritus of Paros, 107
Agrigento, 165
Agriphon, 123
Agrippa, 121, 225
Agrippina, 137
Ajax, 43, 157, 203
Albanians, 87
Alcaeus, 179
Alcestis, 180
Alciati, 27, 91, 194, 196, 225
Alcibiades, 113
Alcides, 43, 59
Alcina, 44, 57, 200
Alcmaeon, 158
Alcmene, 179, 181
Alessandro I, Duke, 170
Alexander, 55, 61, 113–14, 117–18, 145, 204
Alexandria, 56
Alienum, 72
Alipedis, 123
Allah, 122
Alphonso I, 106
Altomare, Donato, 55–56, 62–63
Amaltheia, 64
Amarulentia, 175
Amasis, King of Egypt, 147
Amazons, 69, 180
Ambianus, 77
Ambrose, Saint, 72
Amentia, 77
Ammon, 65
Amphiaraus, 158
Amphistides, 93
Amphitryon, 181
Amphrysus, 69
Amyntor, 37

Amythaon, 38
Anacroia, 217
Andabates, 47
Andreuccio of Marano, 98
Androgeos, 37
Andronica Rodiana, 195
Angelica, 44
Angelucci, Teodoro, 201, 203, 205, 207, 209, 217, 219, 221, 223
Antaeus, 180
Anthony, Philip, 100
Antigone, 115, 132, 165
Antioch, 116
Antiochus, 110, 117
Antonello da Rubio, 161
Anxurus, 65
Aonia, 217
Aonius of Aonia, 151
Apennines, 179
Aphrodite Urania, 174
Apion, 116
Apis, 87, 158
Apollo, 37, 42, 45–46, 49, 69–70, 80, 102, 115, 123, 127
Apollodorus, 37–38, 46, 87, 115, 118, 121
Apollonius of Tyana, 74
Apostate, Julian the, 165
Arachne, 115
Arcadia, 74, 123, 180, 184
Arcangelo, Santo, 98
Archimedes, 52, 114
Ares, 45
Aretias, 180
Aretino, 175
Argalia, 144
Argives, 45
Argos, 38, 49, 123
Argus, 45
Ariadne, 38, 57, 73, 144, 194
Ariosto, Ludovico, 11, 41, 44, 105–7, 139, 154, 157–58, 204, 214
Aristo, 95
Aristo of Ephesus, 134
Aristogeiton, 98
Aristophanes, 82, 85, 97, 113, 149, 225
Aristotle, 41, 73, 79, 113, 133, 177, 189

arrogance, 115, 147, 183
Artemis, 115
Artemon, 81
Arvernians, 114
Ascanius, 116
Asclepiades of Prusa, 37
Asclepius, 37
Ascoli, Ciecco d', 130
Asinius, 215
Asopus, River, 107
Assabinus, 65
Assyrians, 87, 109, 138
Astolfo, 44, 158, 160
Astyages, 47
Atabyrius, 65
Athamas, 158
Athanaric, 185
Athena, 27
Athenaeus, 71–72, 74, 109–10, 116–17, 133, 138, 143, 145–47, 159, 215
Athens, 146, 156, 161, 174, 221, 225
Atlante, 38, 44
Atlas, 62, 123, 180
Attean Virgin, 59
Atticus, 79
Attila, 184–85
Augeas, 180
Augustus, 142
Aulus Gellius, 118, 163, 177
Aurelius, Marcus, 112
Ausonius, 48, 132, 153
Avvi, 185

B

Babylon, 50, 214
Baccano, 86
Bacchae, 191
Bacchantes, 151
Bacchus, 30, 42–43, 73–74, 111, 150–51, 159, 191, 218
Bagnacavallo, 36, 63, 100, 159
Baiardo, 73
Barlachia, 10
Bartolo of Calepio, 12, 95
Basel, 49, 56, 134, 138, 185

Bassaris, 151
Bastiano of Monselice, 10, 94
Battista Pio, 37
Bebbe, Parson of, 86
Belfagor, 105
Belforte, 201
Bellerophon, 69, 203
Bellona, 160
Belus, 50
Benevento, 150, 191
Bergamo, 48, 52, 57–58, 79, 82, 86, 95, 197
Bergion, 180
Bernia, 175, 211, 217
Berossus, 214
Bertazzuolo, 63
Biberius, 73
Bimater, 151
Binasco, 73
Biondo, 138, 142, 185
Bishop of Antioch, 116
Bithynia, 37, 89
Black Sea, 47
Boccafresca, 147, 197
Boeotia, 69, 89, 103, 217
Boians, 116
Bologna, 36–37, 85, 98, 100, 118, 179
    Emperor of, 162
Bona Dea, 119, 190
Bordeaux, 48
Borgia, Cesare, 166
Bormius, 151
Bracciano, 155
Bradamante, 139
Brenta River, 58, 86–87
Brescia, 48, 86
Brisaeus, 151
Brisighella, 159
Britannione, 85
Brocardo, 99
Bromius, 74, 151
Bronte, 71, 166
Brutus, 78, 149
Bubano, 90
Bubona, 95–96, 175
Bucentoro, 57–58, 86
Bufalo, 90

Bull of Memphis, 87
Buona, 190
Buovio, 217
Burchiello, 175, 211, 217
Busiris, 165, 180

C

Caballinia, Fountain, 69
Cadmus, 45
Caeneus, 48
Caius Princeps, 117
Calabria, 74
Calcabrino, 183, 200
Caldius, 74
Calentius, 131
Calepio, 95
Calidonia da Eppi, 199
Caligula, 117, 161
Callimedon, 146
Calpe, 180
Calubrino, 183, 200
Calvisius Sabinus, 78
Cambles, 159
Cambyses, 158
Camerarius, 193, 196
Camerino, 193
Camestres, 99
Camillus, 123
Cappadocia, King of, 52
Carafulla, 147
Carthage, 118, 132
Casoni, Guido, 2, 211
Cassandra, 78
Cassiodorus, 146
Cassiopeia, 115
Castel San Piero, 118
Castellina, 94
Castor, 51
Castrensis, 119
Castrone, 91
Castruccio of Rovigo, 86
Cataon, 70
Catiline, 169, 231
Cato, 43, 98, 121, 166, 215
Catullus, 78

Cauccio of San Lupidio, 68
Cecrops, 181
Celio, 18, 49, 57, 62, 74, 77–78, 89, 93, 97, 105, 109, 122, 133, 138–39, 159, 161
Celts, 114
Centaurs, 37, 180
Cepheus, 115
Cephissodorus, 146
Cephissus, 103
Ceretani, 58
Cermisone, Antonio, 86
Cesco, 146
Cesena, 102
Chaerephon, 142–43
Charisophus, 145
Charles V, 50, 150
Charon, 42, 79–80
Cheilon, 163
Cheiron, 37
Chimaera, 12, 45, 69, 203
Chioggia, 63
Christ, 74, 165, 189
Cicero, 78, 81, 93, 101, 149, 169, 215
Cimmeria, 67
Cinthus, 70
Cipius, 101
Clarius, 70
Claudius, Emperor, 74, 116, 137
Clearchus, 215
Cleisophus, 145
Cleomedes, 105, 214
Cleopatra, 131, 199
Clisophus, 145
Clytemnestra, 159
Cocai, Merlin, 43, 218
Cocytus, 80
Columbino, 82
Colophon, 70
Comis, 149
Commodus, 112, 129, 142
Constantinople, 62, 116
Corebus, 45
Corinthians, 133, 189
Corio, 138, 143, 185
Coroebus, 78, 97, 214

Corybantes, 207
Corydon, 46, 126
Cos, 37, 180
Cotys, 153
Crassus, 37
Cratides, 96, 134
Cremona, 119, 154
Creon, 132, 165
Crete, 37, 46–47, 82, 146, 167, 171
Critobulus, 37
Croesus, 129
Ctesias, 109
Cuccagna, 73
Cuckoos, King of, 178
Cumean Sibyl, 64
Cupid, 42, 111, 134
Cupra, 119
Cupramarittima, 119
Curetes, 64
Curio, 78
Cybele, 207
Cyclopes, 71, 144
Cyclops, 69
Cycnus, 181
Cyllaeus, 70
Cyllenius, 123
Cyllopodius, 144
Cynethius, 65
Cynthius, 70
Cyparissus, 134
Cypra, 119
Cypria, 121
Cyprus, 135
Cyrrhaeus, 70
Cyrrhea, 70
Cyzicenians, 80
Cyzicus, 80

D

Dabitis, 99
Damasippius, 161
Dante, 68, 72, 167, 183, 200–1, 208
Darapti, 99
Dardan, 133
Darii, 99

Darius, King, 99
Datisi, 99
Dead Sea, 105
Dedalio, 115
Degmenus, 180
Deinias, 146
Deipnosophists, 71–72, 74, 109–10, 116–17, 141, 143, 145–47, 215
Delos, 70
Delphi, 70, 147, 184
Delphians, 91
Demades, 113–14
Democritus, 112, 162
Demophoon, 133
Demosthenes, 146
Deucalion, 115
Diana, 115, 118, 126–27
Dictaeus, 65
Dido, 132–33
Dindymene, 207
Diodorus, 151
Diogenes Laertius, 67, 118, 141
Diogenes of Sinope, 204
Diogenianus, 67
Diomedes, 167, 180
Dionysius, 71, 145, 165, 185
Dis, 83, 167, 171, 186
Disamis, 99
Dithyrambus, 151
Dodonaeus, 65
Doge, 57
Doglio, 25–26, 231
Domenicone of Guastalla, 160
Domestica, 48
Domicilia, 27, 194
Domicilia Feronia, 27, 194
Domiduca, 119
Dominican, 94
Domitian, 116, 117
Doralice, 154
Doriplorus, 133
Dorotea, 21, 232
drunkenness, 29–30, 42, 71–75, 111, 191
Dryopës, 47
Duns Scotus, 43, 130
Durindana, 144

E

Egnazio, Battista, 85
Egypt, 42, 49–50, 87, 91, 107, 118, 124, 131, 147, 165, 180–81
 King of, 49, 147, 165, 178, 180
Egyptian Ox, 87
Egyptian Zeus, 50
Elagabalus, 110, 112
Eleus, 65
Eleutherius, 65
Elia, 72, 225
Elis, 174, 180
Elisa, 132
Empedocles, 118, 203
Enaesimus, 65
Ep, 78
Epaphus, 50
Ephesus, 95, 118, 127
Epimenides, 67
Erasmus, 52, 58, 60, 62, 67, 78, 80–83, 85, 89, 94, 97, 101, 129, 197–98
Erebus, 186
Erinyes, 155, 198
Eriphyle, 158
Erminia of Bohemia, 28
Erymanthus, 180
Erythibius, 69
Ethiopia, 48
Etna, 183
Etruscans, 119, 184
Euboea, 181
Eumenid, 156
Europa, 65, 82, 167
Europe, 32, 86, 119
Eurynome, 144
Eurypylus, King, 180
Eurystheus, 180
Eurytus, 181
Eusebius, 116–17, 138
Eustathius, 78, 97
Eutropius, 117
Evarice, 185
Ewe, 91
Ezzelino, 138, 165

F

Fabulanus, 42, 147–48
Fabulinus, 148
Falopia, Gabriele, 100
Fantis, Antonio de, 130
Farfarello, 183
Fatuellus, 42, 100
fatuous, 48, 97, 99–100
Faunus, 139
Faventa, 159
Februa, 119
Februata, 119
Felapton, 99
Fermo, 85
Fernel, Jean, 12–14, 17, 56, 77, 225, 236
Ferrara, 1–2, 4, 6, 13, 19, 36, 85, 91, 125, 155, 179
    Duke of, 106
Festino, 99
Fidentio, 221
Filisca, Armolia, 200
Fioravanti, Leonardo, 4, 52, 218
Flanders, 214
Flavia Drusilla, 24, 28, 194
Florence, 10–11, 16, 21, 26, 29, 86, 94, 147, 167, 170, 178–79, 221
Foligno, 79
Forli, 91, 100, 138, 159
Fornaretto, 16, 63
France, 150, 170, 185
Franceschino of Montecuculo, 94
Francino of Matelica, 89
Francolino, 125, 155
Frenatrix Minerva, 59
Frisesomorum, 99
Frusina, 86
Frustone, Monte, 155
Fulvia, 169
Fulvius, 96, 134

G

Gabrina, 57, 106, 194, 200
Gades islands of Spain, 180
Gaius Asinius Pollio, 215
Gaius Lucilius, 101
Galana, 114
Galba, 6, 146
Galeazzo, 134
Galen, 12–14, 17, 20, 37, 55–56, 61–63, 77, 116, 166
Gallus Vibius, 122
Gambacorta, 174
Gamphasantes, 81
Ganamantes, 81
Ganymede, 65, 110
Garbinello, 6, 122
Garda, Lake, 154
Gaul, 116
Ge, 45, 102
Geber, 51
Gellius, 149. *See also* Aulus Gellius
Genoa, 166
Genseric, 185
Geryon, 45
Giaches, 221
Giacoma of Piangipane, 198
Giacomo of Pozzuolo, 98
Giorgio Sanese, 171
Giovio, 194
Giraldi, 33, 59, 64, 69, 74, 100, 111, 119, 127, 143–44, 151, 175, 179
Glaucopis, 59
Gnatho, 212
God, 100, 111, 116–17, 123, 174, 189, 201, 217
Gonella, 10, 147, 176, 197
Goths, 185
Gradella, 44, 112, 218
Grandisca, 178
Gratian, 48, 72
Gravallone, 58
Graziano, doctor, 43, 52, 97, 122
Greece, 163, 174, 179–80
Gualdo, 91
Guastalla, 160
Gubbio, 178
Gyges, 129

H

Hades, 83, 171
Hadrian, 142
Haemon of Thebes, 132
Hanno, 118
Harpagus, 47
Harpies, 186
Hecate, 42, 127
Hector, 144
Hegesander, 145
Helicon, 69
Hell, 64, 171, 180–81, 184, 186
Heraclitus, 112
Hercules, 41–43, 45–46, 83, 117, 131, 157, 179–81, 203, 214
Hermes, 123
Hermione, 144
Hermippus, 133
Herodes, Tiberius Claudius Atticus, 79
Herodotus, 47–48, 71–72, 81, 109, 129, 133–34, 147, 158, 214
Herostratus, 118
Hesiod, 78, 173
Hesione, 46, 180
Hesperia, 45
Hesperides, 45, 181
Hieronymus, 165
Hippocrates, 37, 46, 61
Hippocrene, 69
Hippolochus of Macedon, 146
Hippolyte, 180
Hippolytus, 37, 47, 132
Hippona, 42, 134, 175
Homer, 67, 78, 82, 97, 109, 121, 181, 203
Honorius, Emperor, 157
Horace, 18, 73, 78, 89, 101, 149, 153
Hospitalaria, 119
Huguenots, 185–86
Hungary, 192
Huns, 185
Hydra, 11, 44, 179, 181, 183
Hyginus, 121

I

India, 114, 151, 198–99
Io, 50
Iobates, 203
Iole, 181
Ionia, 59, 70
Iphicles, 181
Ira, 142
Isabella, 107, 154
Isaurians, 68
Ithaca, 21

J

Janus, 42, 139
Jason, 83
Jehosaphat, 101
Jerome, 233
Jesus, 7
Jews, 7, 16, 63–64, 79, 172, 193, 234–35
Jocasta, 132
Jodocus, 226
Joel, 101
John, Pope XXVI, 99
Jove, 36, 64–65, 114, 116, 123; *see also* Jupiter
Juno, 42, 64, 90, 115, 119–20, 160, 179–81
Jupiter, 39, 42, 64–65, 82, 103, 111, 117, 123, 151, 160, 167, 171, 179, 183–84, 186, 198
Jupiter Ammon, 117–18
Jupiter Elicius, 65
Jupiter Hospital, 119
Jupiter Penetrator, 65
Jupiter Stone-worker, 65
Justin, 133–34
Juvenal, 50, 161

L

Labradeus, 65
Lacedemonian Cheilon, 163
Lacinia, 119, 180
Lacinius, 180

Lake Trasimeno, 122
Lake Vico, 49
Lambro, 143
Lampridius, 110
Languedoc, 150
Laomedon, 46, 115, 180
Lapithae, 184
Laprius, 65
Larissenus, 70
Larisseus, 65
Latona, 115, 127
Latronus, 138
Laurentia Giglia, 200
Lavinia, 198
Lea, 52, 235
Learchus, 158
Lebanon, 86
Lemius, 69
Lemnius, 144
Lemnos, 144
Lenaeus, 151, 218
Leo, Pope, 150
Leonio, 178
Lernea, 179
Lethe, 80
Leucadia, 132
Leucadius, 70
Libellus, 63
Liber, 71, 74, 151, 163, 218
Liberus, 74
Libya, 48, 50, 81, 180
Libyssinus, 70
Licinius Mutianus, 49
Ligio, 123
Lioness, 87
Lirone, 94
Livia Veletri, 195
Livorno, 86
Livy, 191
Lizzafusina, 86
Locresians, 74
Logios, 123
Logistilla, 44
Lollianus of Ephesus, 142
Lombards, 138
Lombardy, 190

Lorenzino of Chioggia, 125
Lucan, 114, 159
Lucchino of Fusolara, 95
Lucetia, 119
Lucetius, 65
Lucian, 78, 82, 97
Lucietta da Sutri, 191
Lucilius, 149, 183
Lucilla da Camerino, 28, 193
Lucina, 119
Ludovico il Moro, 170
Lugo, 63
Lyaeus, 73, 74, 191, 218
Lycaeus, 65
Lycaon, 184
Lychion, 115
Lycia, 49, 70
Lycius, 70
Lycurgus, 133
Lycus, 181
Lydia, 129, 131, 159, 181
Lymira, 48–49
Lynceus of Samos, 145–46
Lyndia, 59
Lyons, 55, 59, 71

M

Macedonia, 37, 141
Macedonia, King of, 116–17, 145–46
Machaon, 37
Macrobius, 184
Maestro Grillo, 217
Maffei, Rafaello, 134
Maia, 123
Mainardi, Arlotto, 10
Mainardo, 222
Maleaeus, 65
Mallorca, 229
Mamachutes, 97
Mambrino, 144
Mamertus, 160
Mandiogene, 146
Mandricardo, 144
Maniae, 186
Mansueta Brittania, 30, 196

Mantua, 26, 30, 86, 160, 218
Manuzio, Paolo, 142, 159
Marcella, Claudia, 29, 190
Marche, 165
Marchetto of Piombino, 68
Marchetto of Tolentino, 79
Marchione of Buffalora, 159
Marforio, 175
Marganor, 105
Margherita of Bologna, 193
Margute dal Binasco, 73
Margutte, 110
Mariccus, 116
Marietta, 198
Marinello da Gambacorta, 174
Marinello of Villafranca 13, 100
Marino, 49
Marmarinus, 70
Marostica, 63
Marquisate of Ancona, 119
Mars, 42, 124, 144, 160, 181, 219
Marseilles, 150
Marsyas, 115
Martia Cornelia, 190
Martial, 117, 207
Martino Turriano, 138
Matelica, 89
Mateuccio of Valvasson, 90
Matia, 192
Mattio, 102
Medici, 170
Meditrina, 42
Medusa, 44
Medusea, 59
Megara, 146, 181
Mehmed, 142
Mejía, Pedro, 50
Melampus, 38
Melchior of Rivabassa, 79
Melissa, 133
Melitides, 78, 97, 214
Memphis, 87
Menaechmus, 146
Menalcas, 126
Mendesians, 48
Menecrates, 116

Menega of Valtolina, 192
Menegone of Olmo, 126
Mercury, 42, 46, 123, 181
Merlin, 200
Mero, 74
Meson, 121
Messalla Corvinus, 78
Mestre, 99
Methon, 121
Methone, 145
Mezentius, 183–84
Miagrus, 175
Michelino of Papozze, 111
Midas, 129
Milan, 52, 73, 91, 95, 101, 134, 138, 159, 163, 170–71, 221
Miletus, 177
Minerbio, 85
Minerva, 42, 59, 65, 115, 195
Minos, 37, 42, 82, 167, 171
Minotaur, 45
Minutianus, 138
Mirandola, 178–79
Misenus, 115
Mitrophoros, 151
Moabites, 105
Modena, 200, 221
Mohammed, 122, 178, 207
Moiano, 122
Molza, Francesco Maria, 211
Momus, 173, 225
Monferrato, 82
Mongibello, 186
Monselice, 94
Montecuculo, 94
Montello, 218
Moors, 98, 170
Morgante, 110, 217
Morienus, 51
Moschus of Elis, 74, 173
Mount Aetna, 118
Mount Baldo, 87
Mount Caucasus, 124, 181
Mount Cuckoo, 94
Mount Cyllene, 123
Mount Dindymus, 207

Mount Helicon in Boeotia, 69, 217
Mount Ida, 64
Mount Maenalus, 180
Mount Oeta, 157
Mount Olympus, 14, 180
Mount Parnassus, 69
Mulciber, 144
Murano, 115
Murranus, 115
Muscovite, 155
Muses, 69, 115, 118, 211, 217–18
Mycenae, 46
Mygdon, 78
Mynors, 227
Myra, 49
Mysia, 80, 177

N

Naples, 13, 26, 48, 55, 167
Navarre, 13, 150, 171
Nedusia, 59
Nemean forests, 180
Neptune, 139, 147, 184
Nereids, 115
Nerine, 59
Nero, 74, 110, 117, 133, 137
Neropolis, 117
Nestor, 43
Nestorius, 116
Nicephorius, 65
Nicoletto, 19, 150
Nicoletto of Francolino, 125
Nicoletto of Gattia, 62
Nicoletto of Orvieto, 150
Nicolò, Giovanni, 99
Nicolò of Monte Frustone, 155, 175
Nicomachus, 133
Nicostratus, 147
Niobe, 69, 115
Nomius, 123
Norandino of Savignano, 102
Norsia, 52
North Africa, 185
Nuvolara, 63
Nyctelius, 151
Nyseus, 151

O

Oblivion, Chamber of, 79–80
Oca, 150
Octavia, 137
Odysseus, 97, *see also* Ulysses
Oedipus, 57, 132
Oeta, 157, 203
Oglio, river, 58
Olimpio, 94
Omphale, 131, 181
Operaria, 59
Opigena, 119
Ops, 42, 64, 186
Oratore, 78, 93
Orbilia Beneventana, 191
Orbilius of Benevento, 78
Orceus, 65
Orcus, 149, 186
Oreos, 151
Orestes, 159
Orient, 51
Orpheus, 218
Orsolina Capoana, 192
Ortensia Quintilia, 197
Ortensio of Sarni, 94, 197
Oscus, 173
Osiris, 151
Ostilia of Modena, 200
Ostrogoths, 185
Ottomans, 127, 142
Ovid, 47–48, 50, 68, 71, 115, 127, 131, 134, 138, 157–58, 184
Ox of Egypt, 42

P

Padella, 112
Padoano, 144
Padua, 36, 58, 86, 94, 100, 122, 138
Palamedes, 121
Pallas, 59, 143
Pamphilus Saxus, 133
Pamphylia, 127
Pan, 95, 100
Panompheus, 65
Pantagruel, 73

Pantaleon, 146
Papeus, 65
Papozze, 111
Paracelsus, 52
Paris, 56, 77, 98, 171
Parma, 94
Parnassus, 212
Parson of Bebbe, 86
Parthians, 106
Pasiphaë, 96, 167
Pasquino, 175
Patara, 70
Pataraeus, 70
Paterno, Bernardino, 36–83
Paul, Saint, 58
Paulinus, Saint, 48
Paulus Aegineta, 56, 61
Paulus Aemilius, 141
Paulus Medicus, 17, 56, 61
Pausanias, 174, 180
Pedrala, 218
Pedretto of Moiano, 122
Pedruccio, 111
Pegasus, 57, 69
Peirithous, 83
Penates, 42
Pentheus, 23, 159
Periander, 133
Perseus, 141
Persia, 158, 184, 214
  King of, 158, 184
Persius, 229
Petrarca, 230
Petruccio of Prato, 63
Petulon, 52
Phaedra, 37, 47, 132
Phaestians, 146
Phaestos, 146
Phalaris, 165
Phaon, 132
Pharaoh, 165
Pheidias, 39, 107, 174
Phigalia, 74
Phigalians, 74
Philaemon, 109
Philagros, 142
Philemon, 109

Philetas of Cos, 48
Philip of Macedonia, 37, 116–17, 145–47, 214
Philippides, 163
Philistion of Nicaea, 162
Philologus, 118
Philonides of Malta, 85
Philostratus, 74, 142, 230
Philoxenus, 215
Phineas, 158
Phlegethon, 80
Phlegyas, 184
Phoebus, 67, 69, 212
Phoenicians, 124
Phoenix, 37, 65
Phrandone, 52
Phrygia, 207
Phrygians, 78, 99
Phylarchus, 147
Phylleus, 70
Phyllis, 133
Physiologus, 231
Piacenza, 2, 154, 199, 228
Piangipane, 198
Piantalimone, 52
Piave, 58
Piazza San Marco, 112
Piedmont, 82
Pietra Mala, 126, 179
Pietro Antonio, 160
Pietro Hispano, 99
Pinabello, 194
Pincerna, 218
Pio, 37
Piombino, 68
Piovano Arlotto, 94, 148, 226
Pisa, 36, 86, 233
Pisander, 18, 62
Pistor, 65
Pius, 132
Plato, 50, 203, 230
Pliny, 37, 48–50, 73, 79, 81, 121, 138, 194
Plutarch, 96, 105, 134, 141, 177–78
Pluto, 83, 180, 186
Plutus, 82
Po, river, 58, 86–87, 111, 125, 155, 160
Poene, 45
Polias, 59

Policrates, 165
Policriti, Giuseppe, 38
Poliorcetes, Demetrius, 147
Poliziano, Angelo, 132, 137, 163
Pollio, 142
Pollux, 51
Polycrates, 165
Polynice, 165
Pontano, Giovanni, 48, 134
Populonia, 119
Porcia, 174
Porcius Cato, 43
Pordenone, 174, 178
Pornopius, 69
Portugal, 185
Porzia, 174
Poseidon, 46, 50
Poseidonius, 55
Posidonio, 61
Possevino, 230
Praedator, 65
Prato, 63
Prester John, 86
Preto, 38
Priam, 78
Primus Domitianus, 117
Prometheus, 124, 181
Pronopius, 69
Propertius, 37, 131–32, 158
Proserpine, 83
Prosymna, 119
Protagoras, 50
Proteus, 203
Provence, 150
Prudence, 205
Pseudo-Aristotle, 113, 177
Psyllians, 48
Ptoenphae, 48
Pulci, Luigi, 110, 217–18
Pultrunzon, 52
Pulvereus, 65
Pygmalion, 134
Pyraichmes, 180
Pyramus, 131
Pyrenees, 44
Pyrrho of Elis, 141
Pythagoreans, 189

Q

Queen of Carthage, 132
Queen of Egypt, 131
Queen of Heaven, 119
Queen of Sheba, 195
Quintia Emilia, 28, 198
Quintilian, 78, 116
Quintius Curtius Rufus, 117
Quintius Rutilius, 196
Quintus Curius, 169
Quintus Remnius Palaemon, 116

R

Raimondina, 214
Ramon, 51
Ravenna, 4–6, 9–10, 25, 36, 90, 99, 198
Raymond, 229
Rector of Olympus, 64
Redondo, 6, 234
Remulus Numanus, 116
Revenger of Misdeeds, 186
Rhadamanthus, 42, 82, 171
Rhamnusia, 107
Rhea, 64, 207
Rhemnius Palaemon, 116
Rhodians, 69
Rhynthon, 146
Rialto, 51
Riccio, Pietro, 178
Rimini, 91, 98, 102
Rinaldo, 73, 144
Risius, 42, 111
Ritonda, 111
Rodomonte, 154
Romagna, 90, 98, 114, 167
Romano, Ezzelino da, 165
Rome, 42–43, 50–51, 68–69, 90, 110–11, 114, 141, 147–50, 165, 170
Romeo, 131
Romulus, 105
Rovigno, 49
Rovigo, 111
Rubia, 161
Ruscelli, 170, 211

S

Sabinus, 78
Sagaris, river, 181
Salia, 160
Sallust, 169
Salmoneus, 118, 186
Salverio Orlando, 163
Samnites, 29, 197
Samos, 90, 165
Samosata, 116
San Bonifacio, 111
San Giorgio, 85
San Marco, 86
San Marino in Romagna, 199
San Paolo, 58
Sandrino, 126
Sansovino, Francesco, 142
Santa Anna, 36
Santino of Tripalda, 58
Santuccio of Fermo, 85
Sappho, 132
Sardanapalus, 109, 138
Sarni, 94, 197
Sassoferrato, 94
Satore, 64
Satumiterus, 151
Saturn, 51, 64, 119, 186, 219
Saturnia, 119
Savignano, 102
Scarlino of Viadana, 86
Scarpaccia of Gradisca, 178
Scarperia, 86
Scillutia, 59
Sciras, 59
Scopa, 167
Scotus, 43
Scribonius Curio, 78
Sellus, 118
Semele, 151, 208
Semiramis, 133–34
Sempronia, Martia, 196
Seneca, 47, 57, 68, 78, 138, 142, 158, 173
Sentinius, 42
Sentinus, 82
Serapis, 87
Servitius Vatia, 68

Servius Sulpicius Galba, 146
Sessa, 56
Sesto Nevio, 149
Siena, 199, 226
Silanus, 137
Silius Italicus, 133, 137, 138
Simon, 166
Sinigallia, 68
Sir Grunt, 174
Sir Mattio, 102
Sirius, 203
Sisyphus, 186
Siwa, 118
Smintheus, 70
Socigena, 119
Solomon, 130
Soria, 53
Sosicrates, 146
Sospita, 42
Spain, 180, 185
Sparsus, 57
Sparta, 72
Sporos, 110, 133
Stator, 64
Stellata, 155
Stercutius, 51
Stimele, 191
Strabo, 69
Straparola, 199
Straton, 146
Strozza the Elder, 131, 184
Stygian Lake, 80, 167
Styx, river, 80
Subtilis, Doctor, 43
Suetonius, 110, 117, 133
Sufis, 58
Sulla, 147
Sultan of Egypt, 178
Summanus, 186
Surius, 49
Sutri, 191
Sylvanus, 175
Symbola, 193, 196
Syracuse, 145, 165, 185
Syria, 53, 55, 86, 110, 117
    King of, 110, 117

T

Tacitus, 87, 116–17, 137
Tadia of Pozzuolo, 192
Tagliamento, river, 58
Talpino, 57
Tansillo, Luigi, 211
Tantalus, 186
Tarcagnota, 214
Tarentum, 146
Taro, 160
Tarquinia, 49
Taurus, 127
Telamon, 157
Telephanes of Samos, 146
Teneatus, 70
Teobaldo da Cantiana, 178
Teronia Elvezia, 30, 191
Tesino river, 134
Thebes, 165, 179, 181
Themis, 102–3
Themison of Cyprus, 117
Theodorus Priscianus, 62
Theodosius, 116
Theognetus, 146
Theophrastus, 147
Thersites, 43
Theseus, 37, 83, 133
Thespiades, 179
Thespius, 179
Thetis, 144
Thrace, 133, 153, 180
Thraso, 118
Thrasyllos, 177
Thyestes, 47
Thyon, 151
Thysbe, 131
Tiberius, 73, 116, 162
Ticino, 134
Tilphosius, 70
Timanthes, 137
Timidus Plutus, 82
Timon the Misanthrope, 82
Tiresias, 48
Tirone, 134
Tiryns, 147–48, 179
Tirynthius, 179

Tisiphone, 42, 155–56
Tityos, 186
Tixier, Jean, 47–50, 78, 80–83, 96–98, 109–10, 121–22, 131–34, 137–39, 141–42, 145–47, 157–59, 178–79, 183–85, 215
Togna, 218
Tognazzo Panada, 192
Tolentino, 79
Tonio Buffalora, 90
Tortellio Novarese, 167
Totila, 185
Tralles, Alexander of, 55
Treviso, 38, 218
Tripalda, 58–59
Triphylius, 65
Tristia, 229
Tritonia, 59
Troglodytes, 81, 87
Troy, 46, 97, 180
Trucco, 166
Tullius, Marcus, 149; *see also* Cicero
Turks, 52, 58, 142, 207
Turnus, 116, 139, 184
Tuscan, 118
Tuscany, 21, 159
Tutelaries, 42
Typhis, 83
Tyrians, 133, 181

U

Udine, 178
Ultor, 65
Ulysses, 78, 157, 203, 214
Umbria, 178
Unxia, 119
Uranus, 102–3

V

Vacia, 68
Vagus, 179
Valcamonica, 48, 86
Valentino, 118, 166
Valerius Maximus, 109, 113–14, 185
Valerius Messalla Corvinus, 78

Valtelina, 86
Valtolina, 30, 86, 192
Varese, 159
Varro, Marcus, 146
Varrus of Perge, 118
Vatia, 68
Vedius Pollio, 142
Veletri, 195
Venice, 41, 56–58, 70, 86–87, 95, 123, 133, 142, 144, 170–71
Venilia, 139
Venus, 111, 132, 134, 144, 160, 213
Venusia, Cecilia, 28, 199
Verona, 87, 111
Viadana, 86
Vicenza, 63, 174
Villafranca, 100, 159
Virgil, 47–48, 64, 78, 98–99, 115, 139, 183–84, 196, 198
Visconti, 143
Visigoths, 185

Volsci, 191
Volterra, 223
Volterrano, 134
Voluptina, 162
Vulcan, 42, 143–44, 160

X

Xenophon, 72, 110
Xerxes, 133–34, 184

Z

Zanfardino, 154
Zani, 198
Zante, 22, 75
Zerbino, 107
Zeus, 45, 50, 64, 82, 123, 181
Zeuxis, 39
Zoilus, 215